A DIET YOU CAN LIVE WITH

Dinner Menu, Day 19, on the Maintenance Diet in *How to Control High Blood Pressure Without Drugs:*

½ cup marinated mushrooms
4 ounces lean sirloin steak, broiled
1 sliced onion sauteed in 1 tablespoon oil
1 baked potato
1 cup Broccoli in Buttermilk Dressing*
1 cup raw spinach leaves
1 tablespoon Oil and Vinegar Dressing*
1 slice low-sodium bread
1 teaspoon unsalted margarine
1 slice Applesauce Cake*
or ½ cantaloupe
Coffee or tea (optional)

*Recipe included

How to Control High Blood Pressure Without Drugs

Robert L. Rowan, M.D.

Menus and Recipes Created by
Rita Parsont Wolfson

IVY BOOKS • NEW YORK

This book is not intended as a substitute for the medical advice of physicians. The reader should regularly consult a physician in matters relating to his/her health and particularly with respect to any symptoms that may require diagnosis or medical attention.

Ivy Books
Published by Ballantine Books
Copyright © 1986 by Robert L. Rowan, M.D.

Library of Congress Catalog Card Number: 86-20423

ISBN 0-8041-0144-2

This edition published by arrangement with Charles Scribner's Sons, a Division of The Scribner Book Companies, Inc.

Manufactured in the United States of America

First Ballantine Books Edition: November 1987
Third Printing: March 1990

Contents

List of Tables

Prologue

Everyone wants to feel well, a reasonable expectation for most people. But to accomplish this, too many of us rely too heavily on medications and too little on healthful living. As a physician, I know full well that medicine has its proper and important place—drugs can be life-saving in many situations. However, equally basic, especially to preventive medical care, are proper exercise, diet, and the discontinuance of smoking and use of alcohol.

The intent of this book is not to discourage the use of drugs to care for an ill person. Rather, I am aiming to prevent an overreliance on medications—and their painful side effects—by avoiding the illness in the first place whenever feasible. And I want to minimize the need for possibly harmful drugs by substituting a more healthful life-style.

To better understand the possible dangers of medication, I'd like to list just some of the problems that can result from hypertensive drugs:

- changes in body chemistry
- poisonings
- impotence
- abnormal interaction with other foods and medications
- birth defects.

The amount of medication you take has a direct influence on the complications that may result from a drug. A reducation in the amount of drugs you take will, in general, decrease the potential for problems.

Why not reduce your need for medicines by simply correcting your life-style? It's much easier than you think, and it's all spelled out for you here. So do yourself a great service—live better . . . longer.

I

THE BASICS

~~~~~~

Learning the facts behind the hidden disease called hypertension, an ailment that millions suffer from without even knowing it.

1 〰

How to Tell If You Have Hypertension

Today millions of Americans are victims of hypertension (high blood pressure). Many of them don't know they have the disease, and they won't find out until a major illness such as a heart attack or a stroke occurs.

Because hypertension is often a symptomless disorder, the only sure way to tell if you have it is to see that your blood pressure is checked at least once a year. You are your own first line of defense in the battle against hypertension. If you get nothing else from this book but the stimulus to have your blood pressure taken, you will have received more than your money's worth.

What Is Hypertension?

Hypertension is an abnormal condition in which the blood pressure exceeds the accepted normal reading of 120/80. These numbers refer to the distance in milli-

3

meters that the pressure within your system would push a column of mercury upward. (You may wonder why I talk about millimeters of mercury when you don't see mercury in the instrument used to measure blood pressure. Today most instruments use air pressure equal to that of mercury, although some doctors still use the mercury-style apparatus. Both models are equally dependable.)

The first of the two numbers mentioned (120) refers to the systolic pressure; the second (80), to the diastolic pressure. Your blood pressure, which is rhythmic, is highest when the left ventricle of the heart contracts—at this instant, the heart is said to be in systole. The pressure is lowest when the heart is at rest—when it is in diastole. The diastolic pressure is more significant because it defines the lowest constant pressure on the arteries.

In hypertension, the force exerted by the blood beating against the artery wall is above the level considered normal. Until recently, the National Heart, Lung, and Blood Institute considered a pressure of 160/95 to be hypertension and the range between 140/90 and 160/95 to be borderline hypertension. But these demarcations are very inaccurate, for any sustained rise in pressure is indicative of hypertension and medical observation.

The latest classifications of hypertension are as follows:

- Mild hypertension: 90 to 104 diastolic
- Moderate hypertension: 105 to 114 diastolic
- Severe hypertension: above 114 diastolic

Hypotension—the Other Side of the Coin

Sometimes the blood pressure is below what is considered the normal level. This condition, the opposite of hypertension, is called hypotension. It is commonly seen in patients in shock, although it also can be found to a much lesser degree in healthy, normal people.

It is generally agreed that people who have low blood pressure have a longer life expectancy than others, as there is less wear and tear on the arteries. Because of the lower pressure, the heart also expends less effort.

Many people with low blood pressure have no symptoms at all, and not all physicians agree that such symptoms as fatigue, dizziness, and occasional lightheadedness are caused by hypotension. However, if you do have any of these symptoms, you should have your blood pressure checked.

Understanding Hypertension

To understand what happens when hypertension occurs, picture a garden hose attached to a faucet, through which water flows, watering the lawn. Now place your foot on the hose near its far end. Slowly start applying pressure so that you are cutting down the flow of water within the hose. As you increase the pressure with your foot, the flow decreases and the pressure of the water within the hose starts to rise. Eventually the pressure will cause the hose to rupture, especially if there is a weak area within its walls. This is essentially what happens when the arterioles (the smallest arteries) begin to block the flow of blood, leading to a stroke as the pressure explodes the artery wall.

In hypertension, the arteriole walls thicken, possibly as a result of an increase in the number of muscle cells that compose the walls. We do not yet undersand how this comes about, but it may be due to increased fluid within the cells.

Many experts feel that thickening of the arterial wall follows kidney malfunction, which increases the amount of water retained in the body. For this reason, however, the intake of sodium, which causes the body to retain water, is an important factor in controlling high blood pressure. Because sodium makes up 40 percent of common table salt, many health experts recommend the reduction of salt in your diet, even though the value of low-sodium foods has not been absolutely proven for people who do not suffer from hypertension.

At a recent medical symposium sponsored by the National Kidney Foundation, the Department of Health and Human Services, and the International Life Sciences Institute (an industry group), some experts challenged the idea of reducing salt in a *normal* person's diet. However, it was generally agreed that too much sodium in the diets of people with a predisposition to hypertension was harmful.

You might best express the problem by saying that there are people who have a hypersensitivity to salt, and when they eat too much salt, they become hypertensive.

Who Is Most Likely to Get High Blood Pressure?

Older people are more susceptible than the young, and blacks of every age group have a greater incidence of high blood pressure than whites.

The U.S. Public Health Service study on Health and Nutrition of 1971–74, which studied 17,796 people, indicated that the incidence of hypertension among whites and blacks varied as follows:

- White men: 18.5 per 100 people studied
- White women: 15.7 per 100 people studied
- Black men: 27.8 per 100 people studied
- Black women: 28.6 per 100 people studied

Although age plays an important role in this disease, hypertension can develop in people under twenty. Because normal pressure readings in the young are never as high as those found in adults, young people are considered to have high blood pressure when their pressure exceeds the level that is normal for their particular age group.

Under the age of fifty, hypertension is more common in men than in women. After fifty-five or sixty, it is more likely to strike females than males. However, women tolerate high blood pressure better than men do, and more men than women die from high blood pressure.

There is a definite relationship between hypertension and family history. If one parent has hypertension, there is a better-than-average chance that the children also will have it; if both parents suffer from the disease, the odds are greatly increased.

Conversely, some people seem to inherit an ability

7

to "ward off" hypertension. Since we lack knowledge of how heredity accounts for this seeming immunity, we must assume that environment also plays a part.

In all probability, you inherit a predisposition to develop hypertension but need an environmental factor to trigger it. Prolonged stress or a diet high in salt can trigger high blood pressure. Obesity also can be an important factor.

Certain diseases produce hypertension; for example, kidney disease and various types of tumors can cause high blood pressure. Under certain conditions, pregnancy will also produce hypertension, as will some poisons, such as lead.

High blood pressure is less common in tropical climates. This is probably due less to the climate than to the more relaxed life-styles typical in warmer parts of the world.

Some Symptoms to Be Aware Of

Most often, there are no symptoms to warn of hypertension. Many people with high blood pressure feel every bit as well as those whose pressure is normal. But sometimes certain signs are evident, such as:

- Nosebleeds
- Ringing in the ears
- Dizziness
- Fainting spells
- Morning headaches
- Depression
- Blurred vision
- Urinating at night

- A feeling of tenseness
- Flushing of the face
- Redness of the face

Any one of these may indicate high blood pressure.

These complaints are most commonly found in people in the early stages of high blood pressure, unlike the far more serious symptoms of the disease in its later stages, when the body has been damaged.

Because these physical symptoms are so common, some doctors think they have no connection with high blood pressure. They believe that such symptoms lead people to seek medical aid and that hypertension is then discovered coincidentally during the medical checkup, rather than that these symptoms result from high blood pressure.

However, I believe that high blood pressure generally *is* the cause of these symptoms. I've seen too many patients with these complaints who turn out to have high blood pressure, and I do not believe their presence together is coincidental. Seek medical attention if you have any of these symptoms.

2 〰

A Funny Thing Happens When You Discover You Have High Blood Pressure

Discovering that you have hypertension can have side effects that have absolutely nothing to do with your blood pressure and a great deal to do with you. Depending on your reaction, being told that you have hypertension can be a simple statement of fact or an invitation to a disaster.

How do you think you would respond to being labeled a hypertensive? Clinical experience as well as many studies have shown that this kind of label can have very serious effects. It can cause some people to worry more about their health than is normal or desirable. In others, it has caused a decrease in psychological well-being. In still others, it has interfered with job performance and interfamily relationships. In a few patients, it has even increased the chances of a nervous breakdown.

People often learn during a routine physical examination that they have hypertension, or during an examination to investigate some other complaint. Because they have had no symptoms of hypertension, hearing the diagnosis can come as a shock to them. They may see it as destructive to their self-image. It may conjure up memories of some relative with hypertension who then had a stroke and died. The net effect is instant confrontation with mortality—an anxiety-producing encounter. How can this have happened to me? is a typical refrain.

The Defense Mechanisms People Use

Being labeled a hypertensive may trigger any one of a number of defense mechanisms. Among the ones most commonly observed are:

Denial of reality. Many people protect themselves from the unpleasantness of a situation by simply refusing to acknowledge it.

Compensation. Others try to counterbalance the situation by using extreme means to improve or correct some other factor that has a bearing on the problem.

Displacement. Some blame another person or a specific situation for what has happened to them.

Two Different People, Two Different Reactions

A longtime successful author, Bill was sixty when he learned he had high blood pressure. A man who prided himself on his youthful vitality, he flatly refused to accept this finding, insisting that he felt fine and there was nothing wrong with him. Although his doctor wrote him several times, trying to convince him of the seriousness of his condition, Bill ignored the letters. When the doctor finally reached him by phone and once again explained the situation, Bill's response was unchanged: He steadfastly refused to accept the diagnosis and start on a program of therapy. Six months later, he was brought to the emergency room, the victim of a stroke.

Bill's is a typical case of *denial*. He insisted he felt well and refused to believe that anything could possibly be wrong. Unfortunately, there are many patients like Bill; they refuse to return to the doctor and will not make any changes in their life-style or follow any prescribed medical regimen.

They simply ignore any medical instructions they may have been given to treat their illnesses. This noncompliance is another way of denying reality. A commonly heard complaint is: If I hadn't gone to that doctor in the first place, I wouldn't have found out that I was sick—so I'd be well.

George was both a patient and an old friend of mine. When the diagnosis of essential hypertension (hypertension for which there is no known cause) was confirmed, he embarked at once on a self-help program by joining a health club, exercising there every day, and swimming three times a week. Considering that he had walked no farther than to and from his car prior to the diagnosis, the change was tremendous. He lost a great deal of excess weight and then worked at maintaining the ideal level for his height and build. The change in his dietary habits was equally striking. In the past, I had frequently seen him order foods that were cholesterol-laden and heavily salted. Now he made sure he ate a healthful, nutritionally balanced diet. To dramatize the difference, consider the last time we were out: George ordered a piece of fish and suggested we divide it between us so there would be fewer calories for each of us. George decided to take control of his life and deal with high blood pressure by making changes in his life-style. What he did for himself as a form of *compensation* was remarkable. The reward: His blood pressure has come down, and he says he feels like a new man.

This case is a good example of a concept credited to Sir William Osler, the famed physician who rose to the head of The Johns Hopkins Medical School. Osler said that someone with a chronic illness who is forced to take good care of himself will outlive the healthy person who does not. This concept is especially true for hypertensive patients who respond to their diagnosis by showing self-control and making changes in the way they live.

Whose Fault Is It, Anyway?

Ann developed hypertension at the age of fifty-five. She had a high-pressure job and was constantly complaining to her husband that her boss was killing her. When hypertension was diagnosed, Ann instantly blamed her boss: "If he hadn't given me so much work and applied so much pressure to finish it, I wouldn't have high blood pressure now." Her attitude of *dis-*

13

placement became so intense and all-pervasive that Ann finally had to give up her job.

In the case of Stan, a schoolteacher, his students became the focus for blame. "I got my hypertension from all the anxiety those kids caused me while I was trying to teach them some math." His attitude intensified this feeling, and the slightest provocation would set him off until he, too, had to give up his job.

Both these people blamed an outside force for their problems.

Ken is a physician whose father died of a stroke at an early age. Confronted with a diagnosis of hypertension, Ken, haunted by the fear that he would die as his father had, became completely incapacitated. His response was an extreme reaction but one that does occasionally occur.

When Irene came down with the "flu," she coughed and sneezed so often that her nose began to bleed. When her condition became progressively worse, she went to a doctor, who said her blood pressure was up and suggested Irene have it checked a few more times. After various tests were done, Irene was diagnosed as having essential hypertension. Although Irene insisted that she really felt fine and was not going to be disturbed by the diagnosis, she soon became something of a hypochondriac. Every ache and pain brought her to the office, and she required constant reassurance that she was all right. Medical reassurance is often essential to the emotional stability of the hypertensive patient, as has been shown in a number of studies I'll discuss later.

What happens to highly pressured, high-strung people (the ones known as Type A personalities) when they are labeled hypertensive? I have seen some make a complete reversal of behavior patterns; they stop applying pressure to themselves and sometimes even semiretire. Others become even more driven because they feel time is running short and they will be unable to accomplish what they want to do. People respond to the same stimulus—in this case, being labeled as hypertensive—in totally different ways.

What the Clinical Studies Show

These are personal observations. What do we find when large numbers of people are studied? The possible dangers of being labeled a hypertensive were explored in an editorial in the journal *Lancet* of March 6, 1982. It cited a study in which seventy-one people were told they had hypertension when in fact they did not. These people were thereafter more depressed, more hostile, and felt less fit physically than did a control group who knew their blood pressure was normal.

According to an article by Lorraine A. Macdonald, David Sackett, R. Brian Haynes, and Wayne Taylor entitled "Hypertension: The Effects of Labeling on Behavior,"* results of a 1971 study of steelworkers indicated that the absentee rate was higher in those who were labeled hypertensive than in those who were not. Another study confirmed that the absentee rate associated with hypertensive persons was twice as high as that of nonhypertensives. (In the case of the steelworker study one must bear in mind that in 1971 there were fewer advanced tests and treatments, and the knowledge about hypertensive problems was not as sophisticated as it is today. Consequently, being diagnosed a hypertensive at that time may have had a more severe adverse effect than it would today.)

A number of different studies, using absenteeism as

Quality of Life and Cardiovascular Care. January/February 1985. Vol. 1, No. 3.

the measure for the psychological effects of being labeled a hypertensive, have the following conclusions in common:

1. *Absenteeism* from work is higher among people aware of their hypertension than among nonhypertensives or those who have hypertension but do not know it.

2. *Labeling* itself may be harmful even when no treatment is necessary. In other words, increased absenteeism can be present even though someone is not taking medication. (Therefore, in those who do take medicine for hypertension, any absenteeism from work cannot automatically be attributed to side effects or to changes induced in the person by medication but rather may be due to an emotional factor.)

3. *Certain techniques* in care and treatment can often prevent or reverse this increased absenteeism. For example, I had one patient with moderate hypertension who became very concerned about his illness. Early one morning he called to tell me he had a slight headache and thought he should stay home. I advised him to take two aspirin and go to work, a decision that could have been fraught with danger had I not been very familiar with his medical status. (Headaches sometimes are the forerunner of a stroke, in which case going to work would have been very much the wrong advice.) I had followed this man's blood pressure for a long time, and I was familiar with the medications he was taking. However, I did tell him to come by my office immediately after he left work. When he arrived, a check

of his blood pressure indicated that it was well within the safe limits. He said that the headache had disappeared as soon as he took the aspirin and that he had had no trouble later. As I said earlier, the most basic medical reassurance can often overcome or reduce the fears of hypertensives who are "uptight" about their problem.

Help at Work

All medical care need not be given by a physician. In one study carried out at the workplace, medical support was supplied by nurses and paraprofessionals with a physician as backup. In this study, the diagnosis and treatment of hypertension were accomplished at work with excellent results. There was less absenteeism in the 169 people found to have hypertension, who were treated at work and given emotional support, than in a control group of employees with normal blood pressure.

Although the concept of treating people at their workplace is not new, unfortunately it is not as widely used as it should be. Obviously, people treated at work are less likely to be absent than those treated elsewhere. When someone comes to work and then has a problem, he or she is examined on the spot and, unless it is serious, stays on the job. Workers are sent home only if the problem dictates a need for time off.

Determining the Effects of Labeling

In a study* to determine the effects of labeling, four groups were examined:

*Op. cit.

1. people who were labeled hypertensive and were hypertensive
2. hypertensives who did not know they were hypertensive and who found it out later
3. people who were labeled hypertensive but were not
4. people who knew they did not have hypertension

The people in groups 1 and 3 suffered greater psychological distress than those in groups 2 and 4. Conclusion: Being told you have hypertension causes emotional problems.

People in whom treatment does not control hypertension have more emotional problems than do those who can be successfully treated.

While this is easy to understand, there may be a physical basis as well as a psychological one. When the body calls for a rise in blood pressure, an enzyme called renin is released by the kidneys. Renin works in part by stimulating a division of the nervous system, the sympathetic portion, raising the blood pressure. A feeling of tension may result from this stimulation. About 15 percent of hypertensive patients have noticeably high renin levels. It is possible that this group with high renin levels is more difficult to treat and so tends to have emotional problems as a result of physical tension. However, our knowledge of the exact role of renin in the cause and prolongation of hypertension is very limited.

Determining the effect of labeling on hypertensive persons is important because one needs to know if hypertension can get worse once a person is told that he or she has it. It is particularly tricky in those whose hypertension is so low that medication is not needed or even may be harmful. The doctor's dilemma at this stage is whether it is better not to tell such persons that they have hypertension because telling them may make them worse, or to tell them because they should be under medical care.

Obviously, in people with more severe hypertension, there is no debate. They must be treated, and telling them about their condition is the first step in accomplishing this.

Knowledge Is Power

Learning that you have any disorder can produce emotional reactions. First, it is a threat to life expectancy, an uncomfortable challenge at any age. The possibility that your ability to work and to cope with various things may be decreased can mean a shift in your financial status and way of life. Furthermore, any illness is time-consuming. It means visits to the doctor and, possibly, various kinds of therapy. On this basis alone, a diagnosis of hypertension can produce problems. Then, if antihypertensive medications are called for, there is the potential problem of having to deal with drug-related side effects.

Today, 15 percent of the U.S. population is estimated to have hypertension. Whether you are one of this group or simply someone who wants to try to avoid this disorder, the best preparation for the problem is to learn all you can about it as well as about the forms of treatment and the changes in life-style that will help prevent hypertension from happening to you, or aid in its therapy. Knowledge is power.

3 ≈≈≈

Understanding the Dangers and Causes of High Blood Pressure

Medical research and statistics show that if you have high blood pressure, you will die at an earlier age than someone who does not have the disease. But you can markedly increase your life expectancy if you are treated and your blood pressure is controlled.

What Are the Dangers of This Silent Killer?

Untreated, hypertension can lead to a frightening list of life-threatening disorders: heart failure; angina pectoris; acute myocardial infarction (heart attack); rupture of sections of the heart; aneurysm of the main body artery (the aorta); cerebrovascular accident (stroke); kidney failure; and hardening of the other arteries of the body.

Watching Diastolic Pressure

There is a clear-cut increase in illness and death related to high diastolic pressure. Recent findings show that this also is true for high systolic pressure.

If your diastolic pressure is less than 85mm Hg (of mercury) and you are between ages 50 and 59, your chances of dying are 63 out of 1,000.

When your diastolic pressure is over 104mm Hg in this same age range, the death ratio is increased to 153 per 1,000. The possibility of suffering a stroke at this age is seven times greater in people with a diastolic pressure over 104mm Hg than in those with a diastolic pressure below 85mm Hg. The figures I've noted apply only to people *not* treated for hypertension or to people who are treated but whose pressure remains high.

To further underscore the absolute necessity for treatment, consider the following, which also refers *only* to people who have not received treatment.

- *Labile hypertensives* (people whose diastolic blood pressure ranges from normal to high, then back to normal with readings between 80 to 100mm Hg) have a 90 percent survival rate for the first five years after their condition is discovered.

- *Benign hypertensives* (people with mild hypertension, with diastolic pressure readings greater than 90mm Hg) have a five-year survival rate of 66 percent.

- *Accelerated malignant hypertensives* (those who have severe hypertension, with diastolic blood-pressure readings above 120mm Hg) have only a 5 percent five-year survival rate.

In the past, people who had labile hypertension were considered merely borderline or transient cases. Now we know that even labile hypertension poses an increased risk and frequently can lead to full-blown hypertension. In fact, even a single high pressure reading should be followed by further readings to make sure that serious disease is not developing—and if it does, to insure immediate care.

Systolic Hypertension Can Be Significant

Of course, you cannot define the various levels of hypertension in terms of diastolic pressure alone, with no mention of systolic pressure. What role does systolic pressure play in hypertension?

There are indications that increased systolic pressure causes ill effects similar to those caused by diastolic hypertension. One study found that systolic hypertension causes an increase in brain injury, heart disease, and heart failure.

What exactly constitutes systolic hypertension? The National Heart, Lung, and Blood Institute defines it as a level of systolic pressure of 150mm Hg or higher, with a corresponding diastolic pressure of no more than 90mm Hg.

Strangely enough, we really have no definitive knowledge about the effects of systolic hypertension. In fact, seventeen different medical centers are currently evaluating this problem. The central thrust of their study is to discover whether strokes occur more often in persons with elevated systolic pressure but normal diastolic pressure than in those whose systolic pressure is not elevated, and whether strokes can be prevented if these people are treated with medication.

Until recently doctors assumed that systolic hypertension had no significance. Any rise in systolic pressure was simply considered a response to aging. The difference between systolic and diastolic pressure is called the pulse pressure, a numerical figure that increases with age. The normal pulse pressure is 40— a figure reached by subtracting the normal diastolic pressure (80) from the normal systolic pressure (120).

Effect of Aging on Systolic Pressure

As you age, the systolic pressure rises, so that your pulse pressure increases; for example, a systolic pressure of 140 and a diastolic pressure of 80 equals a pulse pressure of 60—or 20 points above "normal."

What causes the systolic pressure to rise with age? In large part, the rise occurs because the major arteries of the body are affected by arteriosclerosis, or hardening of the arteries. Normally, each time your heart ejects its volume of blood, the major arteries of the body absorb the pressure, and the systolic pressure does not rise above 120mm Hg. As you age, elasticity is lost, so that when the heart ejects its blood volume into the artery, the artery does not expand, and the systolic pressure rises beyond 120mm Hg. We know some factors related to hardening of the arteries, but we do not know the cause. A portion of the seventeen medical centers' study of systolic hypertension is aimed at determining whether the systolic rise in the inelastic artery is a normal response to aging, or a disease process that can and should be treated.

Older people with systolic hypertension can control their disorder with medication, but the response is slow. (Diastolic hypertension appears to respond to treatment even more slowly than does systolic hypertension.) Older patients respond particularly slowly because their bodies take longer to adjust; therefore, older people must receive medication at a slower rate and over a longer period than younger people.

Anxiety and Systolic Pressure

Systolic pressure often responds to anxiety and returns to normal once the anxiety abates. I recently saw an example of this in one of my patients. Before her physical began, her pressure was 120/80. By the time the examination was completed, her blood pressure had risen to 160/80. Since I knew she tended to be an anxious person, I suggested she rest in the office for half an hour. When I rechecked her pressure, it was back to 120/80. Systolic blood pressure tends to be variable in many people, and it returns to normal rapidly. Doctors should always consider the emotional component in dealing with anyone who has systolic hypertension.

Essential Hypertension: Cause Unknown

This book considers the kind of hypertension for which there is no known cause: *essential hypertension*. Essential hypertension accounts for almost 90 percent of all cases of high blood pressure. Of the remaining approximately 10 percent, true kidney disease accounts for 5 percent, renovascular disease (kidney or renal hypertension) for 4 percent, and narrowing of the aorta for 1 percent. The remaining percentage (under 1 percent) results from endocrine disorders or other rare conditions. All these other forms of hypertension are far less common than essential hypertension, and all have the potential of cure with either medicine or surgery. What do we know about these other causes?

Less Common Types of Hypertension

- *True kidney disease.* This is the most common cause of high blood pressure in those who do not have essential hypertension. The kidney itself is diseased, and hypertension is the body's response to this basic disorder. Examples include glomerulonephritis, or Bright's disease, and polycystic disease. At times the diagnosis can be made with a routine medical evaluation, including blood and urine tests. At other times the diagnosis can be made only using the most advanced instruments, such as the sonogram and the CAT scan. The treatment varies; in some patients, medication is adequate; in others, surgery is necessary.

- *Kidney or renovascular causes.* This type of hypertension results from a decrease in blood flow, usually into one kidney but on rare occasions into both kidneys. Each kidney is supplied with blood through a major artery. When this artery is narrowed, there is a decrease in the blood flow into the kidney. Hardening of the arteries or a growthlike thickening of the artery walls can cause the narrowing. When the kidney is confronted by a decrease in blood flow it responds by releasing a chemical called renin, which increases the general blood pressure, thereby attempting to increase the blood flow into the kidney. While the renin causes an elevation of blood pressure, it does not succeed in increasing the blood flow to the kidney. This is due to the original problem, namely the blockage of the blood flow into the kidney.

Generally the diagnosis is made by X rays that demonstrate narrowing within the artery, or by chemical tests that reveal an increase in the renin produced by the kidney in response to the decrease in blood flow. Various other tests may show lessened function: The sick kidney is seen to be functioning less well than the healthy one.

Treatment involves restoration of normal blood flow to the kidney. This can be done by vascular surgery. A new synthetic artery tube is placed alongside the blocked artery, and the blood is bypassed around the blockage, in much the same way that traffic is routed around a stalled car on a highway. In some cases it is not possible to perform this bypass, in which case the kidney must be removed to correct the hypertension.

- *Narrowing of the aorta.* Some hypertension is caused by a narrowing within the aorta, the main artery of the body. As the blood is pumped from the heart, it enters this major artery. However, in this rare condition, instead of being a wide-open tubular structure, the aorta has a narrow area, and the blood cannot get past this area in a free-flowing manner. Consequently this narrowing produces a rise in blood pressure, causing high blood pressure in the upper extremities but not in the lower. Diagnosis is made by demonstrating the narrow area on X ray, and treatment requires surgical removal of the narrowed section.

- *Endocrinal causes.* Glands that produce hormones make up the endocrine system. These hormones are the chemical regulators that control the body's metabolism. When there is an imbalance in the regulator system, there is an overproduction of hormones, which causes an elevation of the blood pressure. For example, when the adrenal gland overproduces the hormone that regulates salt, carbohydrate, and protein metabolism, hypertension results. Only 0.5 percent of hypertensive patients have this type of disorder.

  The adrenal gland can also develop a specific type of tumor that raises the blood pressure. Blood and urine tests as well as X rays can reveal the tumor. Surgical removal of the tumor cures the hypertension.

  A very small percentage of women who use birth-control pills develop hypertension, which is reversible when use of the pills is discontinued. The cause is believed to be endocrinal in origin.

- *Other causes.* Several other miscellaneous causes should be mentioned: Hypertension can result from brain tumors, which cause increased pressure within the head, and also occur because of a rare type of complication of pregnancy called preeclampsia or eclampsia. Eclampsia is a disease occurring at the end of pregnancy in which the blood pressure can rise to 140/90 or often much higher. The result of this marked rise in pressure is severe internal damage to the mother and at times to the fetus. The cause is not known and treatment is extremely difficult and often unsuccessful.

27

THE BASICS

Doctors reach a diagnosis of essential hypertension only after eliminating any of these other possible causes. This book is about essential hypertension and how you can deal with this condition without undue reliance on medications.

4 ~~~

What You Can Do for Yourself

You must be your own first line of defense against hypertension. This chapter will show you how.

In May 1984, *The New York Times* carried a front-page story about new federal government guidelines for the treatment of high blood pressure. Prepared by the National Heart, Lung, and Blood Institute, the recommendations were for greater emphasis on nondrug treatments, such as diet, exercise, and behavior modification. The newspaper reported that such nonmedical therapies were to be "pursued aggressively" in treating the mildest cases of hypertension. For more severe cases, the government experts suggested that nondrug therapies be used as an adjunct in treatment to reduce the quantity of medicines needed.

"We are responding to a lot of underlying concern about the toxicity of antihypertensive drugs and their side effects," said Harriet P. Dustan, director of cardiovascular research at the University of Alabama, who headed the seventeen-member panel recommending the changes.

She added: "There is a growing appreciation of the fact that obesity and hypertension are closely related. You may be able to control mild hypertension with weight reduction. That would be great. And it would be cheap."

It must be pointed out, however, that the experts felt *only* people with the very mildest form of hypertension could rely on nondrug therapy *exclusively.* These are men and women with diastolic blood pressures that fall between 90 and 94mm Hg.

The foremost advantage to nonmedical treatment of high blood pressure is the possibility—and often the probability—of lessened reliance on difficult drugs. Remember, however, that you should never stop taking blood-pressure medications or change your therapy program without consulting your doctor.

The First Step

Taking your own blood pressure can be the first step in taking care of yourself. But keep certain cautionary thoughts in mind:

When you take your blood pressure at home, it will generally be lower than the readings taken in a doctor's office. The lower reading may be due to your being more relaxed at home. However, there is also the possibility that your pressure is lower because the person taking it is not experienced with the procedure and does not recognize the first sounds that accurately measure the rate of blood flow. Also, the inexperienced person may not place the stethoscope exactly in the correct location.

I have a lawyer friend who bought his own blood-pressure equipment and started taking his blood pressure at his office. On one occasion he asked me to check his readings, and I found my readings to be higher than his. A physician or trained medical assistant recognizes the sounds instantly and therefore obtains a higher and more accurate reading than a novice.

On the other hand, Dr. Christopher Cottier and his associates, writing in the *Journal of the American Medical Association*, reported that for patients with labile blood pressure—those whose readings oscillated just above and just below 150/90—self-examination was very successful.

If you decide to take your own blood pressure, discuss the procedure first with your doctor or with a medical paraprofessional. He or she will have helpful advice on how best to proceed.

Avoid the temptation of taking a reading each day. Constantly waiting for results will in itself put a strain on you and perhaps lead to elevation of your blood pressure. I know it would give me anxiety attacks.

Some Tips for Do-It-Yourselfers

Although you may feel that different people march to the beat of a different drummer, the beat of blood pressure is the same for all. You will hear the following sounds when taking your own pressure:

A literal thump, thump, thump (a sudden loud sound as you release the pressure); this is the systolic level. Then another thump, thump, thump (a louder clear sound), followed by a softening; this is just about the level of the diastolic pressure. Then there will be no sound, which is the time of the most accurate reading of your diastolic blood pressure.

THE BASICS

Besides practice, you will need two basic items to measure blood pressure accurately:

1. A sphygmomanometer
2. A stethoscope

Home blood pressure kits are available at many surgical supply stores and drug stores. They include both a sphygmomanometer and a stethoscope, often attached to each other.

The sphygmomanometer has a pressure cuff that you wrap around your arm about one inch above the crease in your skin at the elbow. After you have placed this cuff, force air into it by pumping the rubbery bulb attached to it via a tubing. The small round disk you see is an air-pressure valve, which you can open and close by simple turning. It will require a few moments of experimentation until you are able to fill the cuff comfortably with air and then release it in a slow, controlled manner.

Next you must locate the artery in your forearm from which you will hear the sounds of your blood pressure. This is the brachial artery and is found within the crease of your forearm at the level of the elbow. You find the brachial artery by extending your left arm in front of you and feeling for an area near your elbow, about two inches from the inside part of your arm. Use the second, third, and fourth fingers of your right hand to find this area.

You may have to continue to straighten your left arm to its full length to find the brachial artery. The location must be accurate, for you need to place the end of the stethoscope directly over this artery for accurate reading. Do not apply too much pressure or you will close off the artery, defeating the purpose of the stethoscope. Apply only enough pressure to be able to listen to the artery but not to cut it off.

Place the earpieces of the stethoscope in both ears; note that the ends point upward to match your ear canal. If you put the earpieces in upside down, they will not fit comfortably.

Pump the cuff to a level that completely blocks any sound coming from the artery. Now slowly drop the pressure, about 2 to 3 mm every few seconds; this will require a little practice. The first sounds you hear will tell you the level of the systolic blood pressure. Keep listening, and keep lowering the pressure; you will find that eventually the sounds of the heartbeats will get very soft and then disappear. This is your diastolic level.

A Story with a Moral

Keeping an eye on your blood pressure is one way to head off hypertension, but monitoring your life-style is even more important. Of all the ailments you might contract, hypertension is affected most by your life-style.

John is forty-five years old and has been told by his doctor that he has early hypertension. The diagnosis leaves John unperturbed even though both his parents suffered from hypertension.

After work he usually places his two-hundred-pound body in his car, heading out of the parking lot to face the heavy rush-hour traffic. On the difficult drive home, John's mind dwells on the frustrations of his job. He feels his boss pressures him to work harder and harder, without either appreciation or compensation. John often thinks his job is killing him.

He is a chain-smoker, generally smoking two packs a day. When caught in traffic, he smokes incessantly.

His supper consists mostly of meals at a fast-food restaurant: double French fries, a cheeseburger, two large Cokes. He adds enough salt to bury the fries, topping them with ketchup.

As time goes by, John is troubled by occasional headaches, which he passes off as just part of daily living. Eventually severe nosebleeds send him to a doctor.

A checkup shows his blood pressure is quite high. John is put on medication to control his hypertension but soon has trouble functioning sexually. He blames his new medication and stops taking it. He has his first stroke at forty-six.

Can You See Yourself in This Story?

Do you tend to ignore warnings to be careful? Do you listen to what your doctor tells you and then promptly forget the advice once the bill is paid—particularly if you didn't like what he or she was telling you?

Do you enjoy eating and drinking too much to worry that your weight is slowly mounting?

Do you drive yourself to excel—to do a better job faster than anyone else? Do you worry that others may be gaining on you at work?

Do you go over and over things that annoyed you until you have built up to a real rage? Do you harbor resentment?

Do you read the warnings about smoking and think that they apply to someone else? Or tell yourself that your grandfather smoked two packs a day and lived to be ninety-five?

Do you add salt to everything? Do you crave salted foods and always give in to the craving? Do you ever stop to think about how much salt you are taking in in a day?

Do you deal with symptoms that frighten you by ignoring them in the hope that they will go away?

Do you think that exercise is for jocks and that you get enough for the average person? When you do exert yourself, do you find that you are immediately winded and can't continue?

If your answers have been yes to many or most of these questions, you may find that you are headed on a dangerous course.

High Blood Pressure and Life-style

As the previously cited (and somewhat exaggerated) case history shows, you are not only what you eat but also what you do.

There are a number of things you should do to minimize the chances of getting high blood pressure or to reduce the risks if you already have hypertension.

1. You must develop eating habits that are nutritionally sound, sticking to foods that provide the basic daily requirements of vitamins, minerals, proteins, roughage, fats, and carbohydrates.
2. You must count your calories and keep a careful check on your weight.
3. You must control stress and anxiety, which can do irreparable harm to your body.
4. You need to eliminate or at least greatly reduce your consumption of tobacco and alcohol.
5. You must reduce your salt intake.

6. You must exercise.
7. If you are found to have high blood pressure, you must obtain medical care and follow treatment exactly.

The rest of this book consists of programs for you to follow. They are based on all the nonmedical therapies recommended by the federal government—namely, weight control, salt reduction, alcohol and tobacco restriction, relaxation techniques, exercise, and more.

But before you begin, I again urge you first to talk to your doctor. *Don't embark on self-medication.* You must involve yourself in your own health care, but involvement and participation do not exclude the professional. And that's a trained physician.

II

YOUR DIET OR YOUR LIFE

~~~~~~

Food as medicine—what to eat and what to avoid to help eliminate reliance on traditional drug therapies.

5 ≈≈≈

The Truth About Salt

To salt, or not to salt: That is the question. One (very good) answer was given in the August 6, 1982, *Journal of the American Medical Association*; the article, "Salt and Hypertension," gave the best summation on the subject I've seen to date.

The article noted that many of the millions of hypertensives in the United States could benefit from a reduction in salt intake. The majority of Americans consume excessive amounts of sodium as a matter of course. This is not to suggest that cutting back on salt will cure high blood pressure or even be an adequate treatment for it; but most people with mild hypertension will show a significant reduction in their blood-pressure readings with a reduction in salt intake.

People who need medication to treat their high blood pressure will have a better response to drugs if they use less salt. Others will need less medication if they decrease the amount of salt in their diet.

For people who lose too much potassium as a result of taking diuretics, a reduction in salt will help to reduce the loss of this vital mineral. It is evident that *reducing salt intake is very important for many people.*

Laura's Story

Although Laura has spent most of her professional life as a dietician developing balanced school lunch programs, she paid no attention to her own diet, which was very poor.

She took in massive amounts of salt daily—even she was aware that she loaded it on. When she began to be troubled by persistent nosebleeds, she consulted a physician, but by the time she did so, the bleeding was frighteningly intense. As her physician suspected, the nosebleeds were caused by high blood pressure, and an examination of the way Laura ate led him to recommend that she cut out salt immediately.

Shaken by the severity of her symptoms and by the diagnosis, Laura decided to practice the dietary good health habits she preached daily at school. She placed herself on a 1-g (gram) sodium diet by eliminating salt from the table, using no salt in cooking, and avoiding any foods that had a high sodium content.

She admitted that it wasn't always easy withdrawing from salt—for a while nothing tasted right—but the adjustment to the loss of salt was made easier when she found that her blood pressure was going down. At her last checkup, her blood pressure was back to normal.

How Much Is Enough?

Salt has played a major role in the history of human beings, but in recent years the role has been that of the villain. In 1960, the U.S. Department of the Interior, Bureau of Mines' *Mineral Yearbook* stated that world salt production was 93.2 million short tons; the United States produced about one-third of this amount.

The vastness of this salt production gives one the feeling that whatever is done with salt, it is too much.

So it is with our daily intake. Most people consume between 2,000 and 7,000 mg (milligrams) of salt each day, yet the National Research Council maintains that a safe and adequate daily sodium intake is about 1,100 to 3,300 mg—for adults. To understand the amount of salt this represents, the average teaspoon of table salt contains about 2,000 mg of sodium.

How much is really enough? It is very difficult to determine the exact minimal amount of sodium that the body needs daily to function. After reading and studying many reports, I believe the best estimate is below 500 mg of sodium a day and probably about 230 mg per day—that is, about one-tenth teaspoonful.

Once we are aware that this extremely small amount of salt daily is all the body needs to survive, the amount of salt we actually consume becomes truly astronomical. It seems clear that the excess sodium in our diet contributes to—and in some cases actually causes—the development of high blood pressure. Everyone should cut down on salt.

The salt content of many common foods is astonishingly high. The list on pages 42–50 provides a good overview of the large quantity of salt in the food and drink that most of us consume. For example:

- A 6-oz glass of tomato juice has 659 mg of sodium—almost three times the most basic amount needed daily, and about half of the minimum recommended amount.

Sodium Content of Common Foods

Food Item	Common Measure (Weight, g)	Sodium mg
Beverages (Alcoholic)		
Beer, regular	12-oz can or bottle (360)	18
Beer, light	12-oz can or bottle (360)	14
Brandy	1½ fl oz (45)	1
Gin (86 proof)	1½ fl oz (45)	1
Rum (86 proof)	1½ fl oz (45)	1
Vodka (86 proof)	1½ fl oz (45)	Trace
Whiskey, bourbon, rye, or scotch (86 proof)	1½ fl oz (45)	1
Wine, red domestic	4 fl oz (120)	12
Wine, red imported	4 fl oz (120)	6
Wine, sherry	4 fl oz (120)	14
Wine, white domestic	4 fl oz (120)	19
Wine, white imported	4 fl oz (120)	2
Beverages (Nonalcoholic)		
Apple juice	6 fl oz (180)	4
Coffee, brewed	1 cup—8 fl oz (240)	2
Coffee, instant	1 cup—8 fl oz (240)	1
Cranberry juice cocktail	6 fl oz (180)	3
Grape juice, bottled or canned	6 fl oz (190)	6
Orange juice, fresh	6 fl oz (180)	4
Orange juice, frozen	6 fl oz (186)	4
Pineapple juice	6 fl oz (188)	3
Prune juice	6 fl oz (192)	4
Soft drinks		
Regular	8 fl oz (240)	11
Diet	8 fl oz (240)	29
Club soda	8 fl oz (240)	56
Collins mix	8 fl oz (240)	20
Quinine water (tonic)	8 fl oz (240)	2
Mineral water	8 fl oz (240)	42
Tomato juice	6 fl oz (192)	659
Tea	1 cup—8 fl oz (240)	1
Tea, instant	1 cup—8 fl oz (240)	2
Vegetable juice cocktail	6 fl oz (182)	665
Breads and Crackers		
Biscuit, home recipe	1 biscuit (28)	175
Biscuit, mix, with milk	1 biscuit (28)	272
Bread, French	1 slice (23)	116
Bread, pumpernickel	1 slice (32)	182

Sodium Content of Common Foods

Food Item	Common Measure (Weight, g)	Sodium mg
Bread, rye	1 slice (25)	139
Bread, white	1 slice (25)	114
Bread, whole wheat	1 slice (25)	132
Bread stick, salt coating	1 stick, small (10)	167
Bread stick, without salt coating	1 stick, small (10)	70
Cracker, saltine or soda	1 cracker (3)	35
Cracker, soup or oyster	10 crackers (8)	83
Roll, dinner, brown and serve	1 roll (28)	138
Roll, frankfurter, hamburger	1 roll (40)	202
Roll, hard	1 roll (50)	313
Cereals (Non-Sugar-Coated)		
Bran, all	1 oz—⅓ cup (28)	160
Bran flakes (40%)	1 oz—⅔ cup (28)	265
Corn flakes	1 oz—1 cup (28)	350
Corn Chex	1 oz—1 cup (28)	325
Granola	1 oz—¼ cup (28)	75
Grits, cooked	1 oz—¾ cup (28)	10
Oat flakes	1 oz—⅔ cup (28)	275
Oatmeal, regular, without salt	1 oz—⅓ cup (28)	1
Oatmeal, instant, regular flavor (salt added)	1 oz—¾ cup (28)	252
Rice, Cream of, unsalted	1 oz—¾ cup (28)	10
Rice, puffed	½ oz—1 heaping cup (14)	10
Rice Chex	1 oz—1⅛ cup (28)	275
Rice Krispies	1 oz—1 cup (28)	340
Wheat Chex	1 oz—⅔ cup (28)	240
Wheat, Cream of, regular	1 oz—¾ cup (28)	7
Wheat flakes	1 oz—1 cup (28)	370
Wheat, puffed	½ oz—1 heaping cup (14)	10
Wheat, shredded	1 large biscuit (21)	1
Condiments, Dressings, and Seasonings		
Barbecue sauce	1 tbsp (16)	130
Catsup, tomato	1 tbsp (15)	156
Chili sauce	1 tbsp (17)	227
Mayonnaise	1 tbsp (15)	78
Mustard, prepared	1 tsp (5)	65
Parsley flakes	1 tbsp (4)	2
Pepper, black	1 tsp (2)	1
Salad dressings		
Bleu cheese or Roquefort	1 tbsp (15)	153

Sodium Content of Common Foods

Food Item	Common Measure (Weight, g)	Sodium mg
French	1 tbsp (14)	214
Italian	1 tbsp (15)	116
Russian	1 tbsp (15)	133
Thousand Island	1 tbsp (16)	109
Oil and Vinegar	1 tbsp (15)	Trace
Salt, table	1 tsp (6)	2,325
Soy sauce	1 tbsp (18)	1,029
Sugar, granulated	1 tsp (4)	Trace
Worcestershire sauce	1 tbsp (17)	206

Dairy Products, Eggs, and Margarine

Food Item	Common Measure (Weight, g)	Sodium mg
Butter, regular	1 tbsp (14)	116
Butter, whipped	1 tbsp (9)	74
Butter, unsalted, regular	1 tbsp (14)	2
Cheese, American	1 slice—1 oz (28)	406
Cheese, cheddar	1 oz (28)	176
Cheese, cottage	½ cup (113)	457
Cheese, cream	1 oz (28)	84
Cheese, Parmesan, grated	1 oz (28)	528
Cheese, Swiss	1 oz (28)	74
Cheese, processed spread	1 oz (28)	381
Cream, half and half	1 tbsp (15)	7
Cream, heavy	1 tbsp (15)	6
Cream, sour	1 tbsp (12)	6
Egg, whole	1 medium (50)	69
Egg, white	1 medium (33)	50
Egg, yolk	1 medium (17)	8
Margarine, regular	1 tbsp (14)	133
Margarine, soft, tub	1 tbsp (14)	152
Margarine, unsalted	1 tbsp (14)	1
Milk, buttermilk	8 fl oz (245)	257
Milk, low-fat (2%)	8 fl oz (244)	122
Milk, skim	8 fl oz (245)	126
Milk, whole	8 fl oz (244)	120

Desserts

Food Item	Common Measure (Weight, g)	Sodium mg
Brownies	1 average (20)	50
Cake, angel food	1 slice, ¹⁄₁₂ cake (56)	134
Cake, devil's food, chocolate icing	1 slice, ¹⁄₁₂ cake (67)	120
Cake, pound	1 medium slice (55)	171
Cake, white, white icing	1 slice, ¹⁄₁₂ cake (104)	243

Sodium Content of Common Foods

Food Item	Common Measure (Weight, g)	Sodium mg
Cake, yellow, with caramel icing	1 slice, 1/12 cake (108)	79
Cookies, chocolate chip	1 cookie, medium (11)	35
Cookies, sandwich	1 cookie (10)	40
Cookies, oatmeal	1 cookie (13)	27
Cookies, sugar	1 cookie (26)	108
Cookies, fig	1 bar (14)	48
Cookies, vanilla wafer	1 wafer (4)	9
Cookies, shortbread	1 cookie (8)	29
Gelatin, plain	1/2 cup (120)	60
Ice cream	1 cup (140)	112
Ice milk	1 cup (131)	105
Pie, apple	1 slice, 1/8 pie (71)	208
Pie, banana cream	1 slice, 1/8 pie (66)	90
Pie, blueberry	1 slice, 1/8 pie (71)	163
Pie, cherry	1 slice, 1/8 pie (71)	169
Pie, chocolate cream	1 slice, 1/8 pie (66)	80
Pie, lemon meringue	1 slice, 1/8 pie (105)	296
Pie, mince	1 slice, 1/8 pie (71)	241
Pie, peach	1 slice, 1/8 pie (71)	169
Pie, pecan	1 slice, 1/8 pie (71)	241
Pie, pumpkin	1 slice, 1/8 pie (71)	169
Pudding, bread	1/2 cup (133)	267
Pudding, chocolate, home recipe	1/2 cup (130)	73
Pudding, chocolate, mix	1/2 cup (148)	195
Pudding, rice	1/2 cup (132)	94
Pudding, tapioca	1/2 cup (83)	129
Pudding, vanilla, home recipe	1/2 cup (128)	83
Pudding, vanilla, mix	1/2 cup (148)	200
Sherbet, orange	1 cup (193)	89

Fish and Seafood

Food Item	Common Measure (Weight, g)	Sodium mg
Bluefish, broiled or baked with butter	4 oz (114)	117
Clams, raw	4 to 5—3 oz (85)	174
Cod, broiled with butter	4 oz (114)	125
Crabmeat, canned, drained	1 can—4 oz (114)	1,250
Flounder, baked with butter	4 oz (114)	268
Haddock, fried	4 oz (114)	200
Halibut, broiled with butter	4 oz (114)	152
Lobster, boiled, meat only	4 oz (114)	183

Sodium Content of Common Foods

Food Item	Common Measure (Weight, g)	Sodium mg
Oysters, fresh	6 small—2 oz (58)	75
Salmon, broiled or baked with butter	4 oz (114)	133
Sardines, drained	1 can—3¼ oz (92)	598
Scallops, bay, steamed	10 to 12—4 oz (114)	302
Shrimp, raw	10 jumbo—3 oz (85)	137
Tuna, chunk, canned in oil, drained	1 can—3¼ oz (92)	328
Tuna, chunk, canned in water, drained	1 can—3¼ oz (92)	312
Fruits		
Apple	1 medium (138)	2
Applesauce, sweetened	½ cup (125)	3
Apricots, canned, syrup	½ cup (129)	13
Apricots, dried	5 halves, medium (24)	2
Banana	1 medium (119)	2
Blackberries	½ cup (72)	1
Blueberries	½ cup (72)	1
Cantaloupe	½ melon (272)	24
Cherries, sweet, whole	1 cup (130)	2
Cherries, canned	1 cup (257)	10
Fruit cocktail, canned in syrup	1 cup (255)	15
Fruit cocktail, canned in water	1 cup (255)	15
Grapefruit	½ grapefruit (120)	1
Grapefruit, canned	½ cup (127)	2
Grapes	10 grapes (50)	1
Honeydew	⅙ melon (298)	28
Orange	1 medium (131)	1
Peach, skinned	1 medium (100)	1
Peach, canned, syrup	½ cup (128)	8
Peaches, canned, water	½ cup (128)	8
Pear	1 medium (168)	1
Pears, canned, syrup	½ cup (128)	8
Pears, canned, water	½ cup (128)	8
Pineapple, fresh	1 cup (135)	1
Pineapple, canned, syrup	1 cup (255)	4
Pineapple, canned, water	1 cup (246)	4
Plums	10 plums (66)	1
Plums, canned, water	1 cup (256)	10
Prunes, cooked	½ cup (107)	4
Prunes, dried	5 prunes (43)	2
Raisins	¼ cup, packed (36)	4

Sodium Content of Common Foods

Food Item	Common Measure (Weight, g)	Sodium mg
Rhubarb, cooked, sweetened	½ cup (135)	3
Strawberries	½ cup (75)	1
Strawberries, frozen, sweetened	½ cup (128)	1
Watermelon	1/16 melon (426)	8
Meat and Poultry		
Bacon, regular	2 slices—½ oz. (14)	274
Bacon, Canadian	1 slice—1 oz (28)	394
Bologna	1 slice (22)	224
Beef, corned	2 slices—3 oz (80)	802
Beef, dried, creamed	1 cup (245)	1,754
Beef, ground, lean	1 patty—4 oz (114)	76
Beef, lean, rump roast	2 slices—4 oz (114)	74
Beef, lean, round steak	6 oz (170)	180
Chicken, broiler	¼ chicken (147)	58
Chicken, roasted	½ breast (98)	69
Chicken, fried	1 drumstick (56)	49
Frankfurter, all meat	1 frankfurter (57)	639
Ham, cured, lean	2 slices—4 oz (114)	1,494
Ham, cured, country, lean	2 slices—4 oz (144)	980
Ham, fresh, lean	2 slices—4 oz (114)	79
Ham, chopped lunchmeat	1 slice (21)	288
Ham, deviled	1 oz (28)	253
Lamb, loin chop, lean	2 chops—4 oz (114)	79
Lamb, leg, lean	2 slices—4 oz (114)	78
Liver, calf, fried	3 slices—4 oz (114)	133
Liver, chicken, simmered	5 livers—4 oz (114)	56
Liverwurst (braunschweiger)	1 slice (28)	324
Pork, loin roast, lean	1 slice—4 oz (114)	93
Salami, dry, beef and pork	1 slice (10)	226
Salami, cooked, beef and pork	1 slice (22)	255
Sausage, pork	1 link (13)	168
Sausage, pork	1 patty—2 oz (57)	259
Thuringer (summer sausage)	1 slice (22)	320
Turkey, dark meat	3 slices—4 oz (114)	91
Turkey, light meat	3 slices—4 oz (114)	61
Turkey, roll	1 oz (28)	166
Veal, cutlet, loin	1 cutlet—4 oz (114)	93
Pasta		
Macaroni, plain, cooked	1 cup (140)	2
Macaroni with cheese	1 cup (200)	1,086

Sodium Content of Common Foods

Food Item	Common Measure (Weight, g)	Sodium mg
Pizza with cheese	1 slice—2 oz (57)	380
Pizza with sausage	1 slice—2 oz (57)	335
Spaghetti, with tomato sauce and cheese	1 cup (250)	955
Spaghetti, with tomato sauce, meatballs, and cheese	1 cup (248)	1,009

Soups, Commercial Varieties, Condensed (Prepared with Addition of Equal Volumes of Water, Unless Noted)

Bean	1 cup (250)	1,008
Beef broth	1 cup (241)	1,152
Chicken, cream of (with milk)	1 cup (245)	1,054
Chicken noodle	1 cup (240)	1,107
Chicken with rice	1 cup (241)	814
Clam chowder, Manhattan	1 cup (244)	938
Clam chowder, New England (with milk)	1 cup (248)	992
Minestrone	1 cup (241)	911
Mushroom, cream of (with milk)	1 cup (248)	992
Onion	1 cup (240)	1,051
Pea, green	1 cup (250)	987
Tomato	1 cup (245)	872
Tomato, cream of (with milk)	1 cup (250)	932
Turkey noodle	1 cup (240)	998
Vegetable beef	1 cup (245)	957
Vegetarian vegetable	1 cup (245)	823

Vegetables (Considered Fresh, Unless Listed Otherwise; Considered Cooked, Unless Indicated as Raw. Sodium Content of Cooked Vegetables Is Content Before Salt Is Added)

Artichoke	1 bud (120)	36
Asparagus	4 spears (60)	4
Asparagus, canned	4 spears (80)	298
Beans, baked, canned, with pork and tomato sauce	½ cup (145)	464
Beans, baked, canned, with pork and molasses sauce	½ cup (145)	303
Beans, green	½ cup (63)	3
Beans, green, canned	½ cup (65)	319
Beans, green, frozen	½ cup (68)	1
Beans, lima	½ cup (85)	1
Beans, lima, canned	½ cup (85)	228

Sodium Content of Common Foods

Food Item	Common Measure (Weight, g)	Sodium mg
Beans, lima, frozen	½ cup (85)	64
Beets	½ cup (85)	37
Beets, canned	½ cup (85)	240
Broccoli	1 stalk, medium (151)	18
Broccoli, frozen	½ cup (94)	18
Brussels sprouts	4 sprouts (84)	8
Brussels sprouts, frozen	½ cup (77)	8
Cabbage	½ cup (72)	8
Cabbage, raw	½ cup (35)	4
Carrots	½ cup (78)	26
Carrots, frozen	½ cup (113)	52
Carrots, raw	1 medium (72)	34
Cauliflower	½ cup (63)	6
Cauliflower, frozen	½ cup (90)	9
Cauliflower, raw	½ cup (58)	8
Celery, raw	1 stalk (20)	25
Corn	1 ear (140)	1
Corn, canned, creamed	½ cup (128)	336
Corn, canned, whole kernel	½ cup (83)	192
Cucumber, raw	6 large slices (28)	2
Lettuce, head, raw	¼ head (135)	12
Lettuce, leaf, raw	1 cup (55)	5
Mushrooms	½ cup (35)	4
Okra	5 pods (53)	1
Onions, green, raw, with tops	2 medium (30)	2
Onions, raw	1 tbsp (10)	1
Peas, green	½ cup (80)	1
Peas, green, canned	½ cup (85)	247
Peas, green, frozen	½ cup (85)	106
Peppers, sweet	½ cup (75)	13
Pickles, dill	1 spear (30)	232
Pickles, sweet gherkin	1 whole pickle (15)	128
Potato, baked or boiled	1 medium (156)	5
Potatoes, french-fried, unsalted	10 strips (50)	15
Potatoes, mashed, milk and salt added	1 cup (210)	632
Radishes, raw	5 medium (18)	8
Sauerkraut	½ cup (235)	777
Spinach, canned	½ cup (103)	455
Spinach, frozen	½ cup (50)	78
Spinach, raw	½ cup (55)	25
Squash, summer	½ cup (105)	3

Sodium Content of Common Foods

Food Item	Common Measure (Weight, g)	Sodium mg
Sweet potato, boiled	1 medium (132)	20
Sweet potato, canned	1 medium (100)	48
Tomato, raw	1 medium (123)	14
Tomatoes, canned	½ cup (120)	195
Snacks		
Caramels, plain or chocolate	1 oz (28)	74
Candy, milk chocolate	1 oz (28)	28
Corn chips, regular	1 oz (28)	231
Doughnuts, cake type, plain	1 doughnut (32)	160
Mints, chocolate-coated	1 small (11)	20
Nuts, cashews, dry-roasted, salted	4 tbsp—1 oz (28)	150
Peanut butter	1 tbsp—1 oz (16)	81
Peanuts, dry-roasted, salted	4 tbsp—1 oz (28)	123
Peanuts, roasted in oil, unsalted	4 tbsp—1 oz (28)	1
Popcorn, salted, with butter	1 cup (9)	175
Popcorn, unsalted	1 cup (6)	1
Potato chips	14 chips—1 oz (28)	285
Pretzels, regular twist	5 pretzels—½ oz (14)	505

- When you put one tablespoon of chili sauce on your hamburger, you add 227 mg of sodium.

- Drench your sushi in a tablespoon of soy sauce and you've taken in 1,029 mg of sodium.

- Have lunch on the run—a frankfurter (639 mg) on a bun (202 mg) with sauerkraut (one-eighth cup equals 179 mg)—and suddenly you've ingested 1,020 mg of sodium. If you add a dill pickle slice you've added 232 mg to bring the total to 1,252 milligrams.

You can see how quickly and easily this mounts up. But once you learn "salt awareness" you can start looking out for your health by cutting back on sodium.

How to Avoid Salt

The first step in avoiding salt is to remove the salt shaker from the table and to keep it off. This may be difficult, but it is essential.

Then try to evaluate the amount of salt you now consume each day. Start a daily salt evaluation chart, listing all the foods you've eaten, the approximate size of each portion, and the amount of salt used with every dish. List everything you ate for every meal: breakfast, lunch, dinner, and snacks, as well as everything you drank.

Now list the medications you are taking; some may be very high in salt. For example, laxatives, cough medications, antibiotics, alkalizers, painkillers, antacids, and sedatives all contain a great deal of sodium. The table that follows lists some of the more common nonprescription drugs with their sodium content.

How to Decrease Your Salt Intake

1. Talk to your family about the importance of decreasing the amount of salt used in cooking. We have all been educated to salt food "to taste," so the reeducation must start by lessening the salt used in home-cooked foods.

2. As noted before, put no salt on the table.

3. Avoid especially salty foods such as potato chips, salted nuts, olives, pickles, soy sauce, corned and dried beef, canned crab meat, ham, and canned soups and vegetables.

4. Reduce the use of processed foods that have a high sodium content. This means reading the

Sodium Content of Selected Nonprescription Drugs

Type of product	Trade Name	Ingredients	Sodium Content mg per dose	Sodium Content mg per 100 ml
Analgesic	(Various)	Aspirin	49	—
Antacid analgesic	Bromo-Seltzer	Acetaminophen Sodium citrate	717	—
	Alka-Seltzer (blue box)	Aspirin Sodium citrate	521	—
Antacid laxative	Sal Hepatica	Sodium bicarbonate Sodium monophydrogen phosphate Sodium citrate	1,000	—
Antacids	Rolaids	Dihydroxy aluminum Sodium carbonate	53	—
	Soda Mint	Sodium bicarbonate	89	—
	Alka-Seltzer Antacid (gold box)	Sodium bicarbonate Potassium bicarbonate Citric acid	276	—
	Brioschi	Sodium bicarbonate Tataric acid Sucrose	710	—
Laxatives	Metamucil Instant Mix	Psyllium Sodium bicarbonate Citric acid	250	—
	Fleet's Enema	Sodium biphosphate Sodium phosphate	250–300 (absorbed)	—
Sleep-aids	Miles Nervine Effervescent	Sodium citrate	544	—
Antacid suspensions	Milk of Magnesia	Magnesium hydroxide	—	10
	Amphogel	Aluminum hydroxide	—	14
	Basalgel	Aluminum carbonate	—	36
	Maalox	Magnesium hydroxide Aluminum carbonate	—	50
	Riopan	Magnesium aluminum complex	—	14
	Mylanta I	Magnesium hydroxide	—	76
	Mylanta II	Aluminum hydroxide Simethicone	—	160 170
	Digel Titralac	Calcium carbonate	—	220

labels on cans and frozen food packages before you buy.

5. Be aware that the following items are really sodium—i.e., salt:

- Baking soda (sodium bicarbonate)
- Baking powder
- Brine (salted water)
- Disodium phosphate—used in foods to aid "quick" cooking, e.g., Quick Cream of Wheat.
- Vegetable salts—the base is sodium chloride with added vegetable extracts, such as celery or onions
- Seasoned salts—vegetable salts, spices, and monosodium glutamate in combination
- Monosodium glutamate (MSG)—a form of sodium usually extracted from grains or beets; it is also present in bean curd and soy sauce and is used to intensify flavor.

Counting Your Salt

If you want a quick and easy gauge of the amount of salt in your daily diet, there is an interesting instrument called a salt meter,* which tells you the level of salt in the food you are eating. Its operation is based on the fact that salt conducts a current of electricity in food; the more salt you have in any dish, the greater the amount of current the meter registers.

---

*Atago Refracto Meter, Stock No. F 34711. Manufactured by Edmund Scientific Co., 101 East Gloucester Pike, Barrington, NJ 08007. Phone (609) 547-3488. Cost, $189.95.

The Real Problem

In some societies salt is a luxury, but not in ours. It is widely available, and an unlimited supply can be had for a small sum. The cheapness and availability of salt are not the basic problem, however. We have to reeducate our taste buds. Salt has a certain addictive quality. As you increase your salt intake, your taste buds become accustomed to the new level of salt concentration; to feel the taste of salt again, you must constantly increase the amount.

We start our salt level as babies. Mother tastes the food and adds salt to *her* taste level, which then becomes the infant's starting taste level. As the child grows older, he or she increases the amount of salt to continue to taste it.

For many years it was thought that people could ingest any amount of salt, within the limits of their taste needs, without ill effect; the body would simply pass the excess salt out of its system. We now know that this is incorrect. Some people respond to excess salt by developing hypertension. Since no one needs salt beyond the very basic daily requirement, everyone should cut down.

For people with any type of hypertension—be it mild or severe—salt intake *must* be reduced.

For severely ill people, salt creates excess strain on the heart, and heart failure can often result from not following a low-salt diet.

What Is Safe?

An adult who makes no unusual demands on his body's salt supply (due to profuse sweating, for example, as a result of exercise) can safely reduce sodium intake to 1,100 to 3,500 mg a day. Although this is considered a "safe" level, it is still quite a bit more salt than is actually good for most of us. It is believed that excess salt is usually passed out of the body, and that people who are salt sensitive develop high blood pressure. If you exercise, you need salt replacement for that lost in sweat. The total amount is very small, however, and the kidneys correct the loss with ease.

The *Federal Register* classifies low-salt diets as follows:

- Mild—2,000 to 3,000 mg of sodium per day
- Moderate—1,000 to 1,500 mg per day
- Severe—500 to 700 mg per day
- Extreme—200 to 300 mg per day

The degree of salt restriction can vary with the level of high blood pressure, the health of your heart, and the state of your kidneys. Consult your doctor before you undertake a severely reduced salt diet.

Sodium-Free, Low-Sodium, Moderately Low-Sodium

Food products should be labeled in a way that will help us control our sodium intake. The guidelines for this labeling must be set by the government, but the *Federal Register* has already suggested the following:

Sodium-free food should be any food with less than 5 mg of sodium per serving. Note that this is *per serving*, not per 100 g of food. The consumer is best served by using this kind of measurement rather than measuring salt on a weight basis. People are more familiar with the size used in a single serving than with the exact amount of, say, 100-g weight.

Low-sodium food should have no more than 35 mg of sodium per serving.

Moderately low-sodium food should contain 140 mg or less of sodium.

What Is "No-Salt Salt"?

Almost every supermarket carries products touted as the "no-salt salt alternative." They promise saltlike flavor without the sodium content. The label says the stuff contains potassium chloride, potassium bitartrate, and other items, and makes its sodium-free claim because it contains less than 10 mg of sodium per 100 g of the product. However, potassium is similar in many ways to sodium. While potassium can produce a taste response similar to that of sodium—salt—potassium has been known to create problems for people with kidney disease. If you have kidney problems, potassium should not be used without a doctor's advice.

Keeping a Low-Sodium House

You may have noticed shelves of no-sodium products in your supermarket—this is a trend that is catching on. A number of salt-free items are available now, and more are coming on the market every day. For one dollar, The Low-Sodium Pantry, 4901 Auburn Avenue, Bethesda, MD 20014, will send you an interesting catalog of low-sodium products, along with excellent ideas for cooking the low-sodium way. Bookstores abound in low-sodium cookbooks for controlling your salt intake while still eating well. A list of these books appears in the Bibliography.

The Spices of Life

As any cook knows, many spices can be substituted for salt to provide flavorings. Here is a short list of everyday spices you can use:

Add Zest with

Herbs

Basil	Marjoram	Sage
Bay leaf	Mint	Savory
Chives	Oregano	Tarragon
Fennel	Rosemary	Thyme

Spices

Allspice	Ginger	Paprika
Cinnamon	Mace	Pepper (black, red
Cloves	Mustard	or white)
Curry	Nutmg	Saffron
		Turmeric

Extracts

Almond	Orange	Strawberry
Lemon	Peppermint	Raspberry
Maple	Rum	Vanilla

Seeds

Anise	Dill	Sesame
Caraway	Poppy seed	

Other

Cocoa (not Dutch process)	Fresh horseradish	Onion
	Leeks	Orange peel
Garlic	Lemon juice	Parsley
Green pepper		Sugar

Beware of Water Softeners

Many water softeners replace unwanted hard-water chemicals with sodium. Drink a glass of water that has

Try These Combinations for Flavor

Meats, poultry, etc.

Chicken: cranberry sauce, ginger, mushrooms (fresh or low-sodium canned), onion, paprika, parsley, sage, tarragon, thyme, tomato

Turkey: cranberries, marjoram, rosemary

Fish: basil, bay leaf, dill, garlic powder, green pepper, lemon juice, majoram, mushrooms, onion, paprika, rosemary, savory, tomato

Beef: basil, bay leaf, dry mustard, garlic powder, green pepper, marjoram, onion, oregano, pepper, sage, thyme, tomato, vinegar

Lamb: cinnamon, curry, dill, garlic (fresh or powder), mint, mint jelly, pineapple rings, rosemary, thyme

Pork: apples, applesauce, caraway, garlic, onion, sage

Eggs: curry, dry mustard, green pepper, jelly, mushrooms, onion, oregano, paprika, parsley, tomato

Veal: bay leaf, currant jelly, curry, garlic powder, ginger, mace, marjoram, mushrooms, onion, oregano, paprika, spiced apricots or peaches

Vegetables

Asparagus: basil, caraway, lemon juice, thyme

Beans, green or wax: basil, dill, lemon juice, nutmeg, onion, oregano, rosemary, savory, sesame seeds (toasted), turmeric, unsalted toasted almonds

Broccoli: basil, lemon juice, oregano, tarragon

Cauliflower: dill, paprika, parsley

Corn: chives, green pepper, tomato

Peas: chives, green pepper, mint, mushrooms, onion

Potatoes: chives, green pepper, mace, onion, paprika, parsley, rosemary

Squash (summer): basil, onion, oregano, pepper *(winter):* brown sugar, cinnamon, ginger, mace

Sweet potatoes: apples, cinnamon, nutmeg, orange juice, sugar (brown and white)

tomatoes: basil, onion, oregano, sage, sugar, vinegar

been through your water softener, and then drink a glass of water that has not gone through the softener. You will be able to taste the salt in the softened water. Although this is a very small amount of sodium, daily use of such water for cooking and drinking can well result in your getting more sodium than you want.

6 ≈

Fat Is a Health Issue

Does obesity cause hypertension? While there is no clear evidence that it does, common sense tells us that a person suffering from hypertension, or one who has a potential for hypertension, is wise not to become overweight. Hypertension is a manifestation of an abnormal vascular system. When you are overweight, you put a strain on your vascular system. Because your body needs a greater food supply to maintain the extra tissue, you need an increased blood flow to meet the metabolic needs of a larger body. If you lose weight, you reduce the need for increased vascular function and heart action. For that reason alone, it makes sense to try to stay thin.

Another way of understanding the dangers of overweight is to consider what would happen if you placed a fifteen-pound weight on your back and kept it there for the entire day. You would find that you needed more energy to get about. Your heart would have to work harder to overcome this extra strain. Being overweight has the identical effect.

YOUR DIET OR YOUR LIFE
The Famous Framingham Study

The small town of Framingham, Mass., was the site of one of the best-known studies on the connection between excess weight and hypertension.

In this study, begun in 1949 and carried on for many years, the people in Framingham who suffered from high blood pressure were found to be considerably heavier than those whose blood-pressure readings were normal. In addition, the incidence of hypertension increased as people put on weight. When people lost weight, their blood pressures went down accordingly. Finally, thin people who had high blood pressure showed a tendency to get fat as their condition continued, further demonstrating the link between weight and hypertension. The Framigham study came to no conclusion as to why people who develop high blood pressure also tend to become obese.

The Life Insurance Study

The lethal role that obesity plays was demonstrated in a study on the relationship between excess weight and mortality rates in a group of 450,000 men and women. The study was conducted by the Society of Actuaries and the Association of Life Insurance Medical Directors, two groups that have access to statistics via life insurance or health insurance records on large numbers of people who have had physical examinations and then whose state of health has been followed for prolonged periods.

The study revealed that when weight was 5 to 15 percent above what was considered normal for the age group, the mortality rate rose 10 percent above the norm for that age. When weight rose to 45 to 55 percent above normal, the death rate was 111 percent above the expected norm. When weight rose to 55 to 65 percent above the normal weight for the age, the death rate rose by 127 percent. The picture these statistics paint is very clear. There can be no doubt that extra weight means a more immediate risk of death.

In clinical practice the relationship between obesity and illness is even more startling. On the brighter side, a decided improvement in a patient's physical condition often occurs as soon as he or she loses weight.

Tom and Jane—a Study in Contrasts

At thirty Tom has had essential hypertension for two years. His problem is compounded by the fact that he weighs 240 pounds, too much for his five-foot, eleven-inch frame. At present he takes two antihypertensive pills a day to keep his blood pressure down. A few months ago he went on a diet and as soon as he started to lose weight his blood pressure went down. By the time he weighed 180 pounds his pressure was normal *without medication*. The minute he began to put weight back on, his pressure went up. He is well aware of his problem since he is a registered nurse and works in a hospital, but unfortunately no amount of reasoning will get him to maintain a desirable weight.

I had a very different experience with a patient I'll call Jane.

Jane was a 5'3" legal secretary who weighed 110 pounds and had normal blood pressure when I first knew her. During the next ten years her weight remained essentially the same, with continuing normal blood pressure. However, when she became an office supervisor, her weight started to climb—along with her blood pressure. Over the next five years her weight rose to 150 pounds, her blood pressure to 150/95. I put her on a strict weight-reduction program primarily to control the seriousness of the pressure elevation. As she lost weight, her blood pressure came down, too. But each time her weight went up, her blood-pressure measurements showed it.

For Jane, obesity and hypertension obviously were related. No one had to motivate her beyond this fact to get her back to her previously thin self and persuade her to stay there.

What I Did for Myself

Being a doctor, I try to keep an eye on my own waist-line. It isn't always easy. But I did get lucky a few years ago, when I shared an office with a psychiatrist. She kept our small refrigerator filled with packages of carrots, celery, lettuce, and melon cut into bite-size pieces. She insisted that when you craved a snack, it was easy to become accustomed to eating these foods rather than cookies, cake, or ice cream, and she was right.

After a period of learning to eat these foods that were good for me, I came to like them. I learned that I could survive on the diet both physically and emotion-ally. After a while I graduated to the point where I could stop at a fruit store, buy an apple, eat it in the park, and consider that to be lunch. If I was still hungry I would have another apple or some other fruit. The change of diet worked wonders for me.

Today I eat a very simple breakfast. Usually I have half a grapefruit (the entire grapefruit if I am hungry) or any other fruit in season. I drink two cups of coffee, both with skim milk, which I have learned to enjoy.

My changeover from a standard hamburger lunch to fruit I consider a minor miracle.

For dinner I start with a large vegetable salad. I find that this fills me up so well that I can limit any main course to an amount that does not have too many calories. Baked potatoes are excellent if you learn to eat them without any sour cream or butter. For dessert the best bets are a simple fruit salad or fresh fruit. Through a process of reeducation of my taste buds I have learned to enjoy only the simplest of foods. I no longer care for anything made with heavy sauces and butter. The diet has not always been easy, but it has been worth it for my health.

I find that it helps to spend some time preparing the meal. I cut salads into very fine pieces, which helps to reduce the volume of the food I eat. To make up for no salt, I bought myself a good-size pepper mill, and I use it freely. Drinking water is also a way to fill up, and although drinking while eating is not ideal, since it dilutes the gastric enzymes needed for digestion, I find that its "filling" quality makes it worth the physiological price.

How Do You Compare?

Check your own weight against those listed in the weight chart. How do you compare? If you are appreciably heavier than the recommended pounds for your age, frame, and sex—beware! Don't be fooled by the assumption that weight means little in your particular case because you, personally, feel just fine. Remember that you can feel great and still have high blood pressure. Hypertension has no symptoms. How you are feeling at the moment doesn't mean that you are not ill.

Desirable Weights (Pounds)*

Men (Ages 25-59)					Women (Ages 25-59)				
Height† Feet	Inches	Small Frame	Medium Frame	Large Frame	Height† Feet	Inches	Small Frame	Medium Frame	Large Frame
5	2	128-134	131-141	138-150	4	10	102-111	109-121	118-131
5	3	130-136	133-143	140-153	4	11	103-113	111-123	120-134
5	4	132-138	135-145	142-156	5	0	104-115	113-126	122-137
5	5	134-140	137-148	144-160	5	1	106-118	115-129	125-140
5	6	136-142	139-151	146-164	5	2	108-121	118-132	128-143
5	7	138-145	142-154	149-168	5	3	111-124	121-135	131-147
5	8	140-148	145-157	152-172	5	4	114-127	124-138	134-151
5	9	142-151	148-160	155-176	5	5	117-130	127-141	137-155
5	10	144-154	151-163	158-180	5	6	120-133	130-144	140-159
5	11	146-157	154-166	161-184	5	7	123-136	133-147	143-163
6	0	149-160	157-170	164-188	5	8	126-139	136-150	146-167
6	1	152-164	160-174	168-192	5	9	129-142	139-153	149-170
6	2	155-168	164-178	172-197	5	10	132-145	142-156	152-173
6	3	158-172	167-182	176-202	5	11	135-148	145-159	155-176
6	4	162-176	171-187	181-207	6	0	138-151	148-162	158-179

*With indoor clothing weighing 5 pounds for men and 3 pounds for women.
†With shoes with 1-inch heels.
Source of basic data: Build Study, 1979. Society of Actuaries and Association of Life Insurance Medical Directors of America, 1980.
Copyright © 1983 by the Metropolitan Life Insurance Company.

Ida is a perfect example of what I mean. Most women her age would have retired, but at sixty-six Ida was still working full time as a beautician and leading an active, busy personal life. Until her early fifties, Ida never weighed more than 135 pounds. At her height— five feet, five inches—that was just fine. But after menopause she began to gain. By her sixties, she weighed 170 pounds.

Now, a lot of people don't go to their physician every year; in fact, latest medical opinion is divided on the advisability of the annual checkup. Ida felt great and had more energy than her thirty-two-year-old daughter. So why bother with the doctor?

But just after her sixty-sixth birthday, Ida came down with flu. (Don't think she bothered with flu shots, either.) It turned out to be a stubborn and unpleasant strain, and when her fever reached 103 degrees, Ida took a cab to her family physician. During a routine check, he found abnormally high blood pressure.

Ida was immediately placed on antihypertensive medication and put on a strict diet. As her weight came down and her pressure fell, she began to need fewer and fewer pills. In fact, as long as she adhered to her diet and watched her intake of salt, she could easily control her hypertension with minimal drugs.

Gain by Losing

Scientific studies back up the points I'm making about obesity based on my personal experience with patients. In 1978, the prestigious *New England Journal of Medicine* reported that weight loss in itself helped lower blood pressure, even in people who were still overweight and even when other measures (such as reducing the salt in the diet) had not been taken. Other research—at the UCLA School of Medicine—showed significant lowering of blood pressure in people who were put on a special twelve-week reducing plan.

How to Get a Grip on Yourself

I hope I've convinced you that overweight can definitely make you ill. So why do you still eat so much when you *know* it's bad for you? I think it works like this:

Eating represents many things to many people, and people eat for many reasons other than simple hunger. If you can understand *why* you eat too much, you can then prepare a program of self-help to overcome the problem.

Do any of these sound familiar?

- I eat because the food is too appealing to stop.
- I eat because I love to eat.
- I eat because I feel I mustn't waste food—I clean up my plate.
- I eat when I'm bored (or depressed, angry, nervous, upset, tired).
- I eat when I'm relaxed and happy and feel like celebrating.

The list is endless, but if you can find and learn to recognize the cause of *your* problem, it will be easier to correct it. I know the process of changing your eating habits is not easy.

Learn to Recognize True Hunger

You should eat *only* when you are hungry. The factors that bring about the sensation of hunger are varied. At first it was believed that hunger pains were caused solely by the contractions of the stomach when it was empty. However, this is only part of the explanation. The blood sugar levels are also a factor in producing hunger. The body needs blood sugar to function, and when blood sugar levels are decreased, there is a desire for food. There are still other, as yet not understood factors that affect the hunger center, which exists in the hypothalamus of the brain. The sensation of hunger arises from this central control.

When we have eaten enough, we have a sense of satiation, and this should be the signal to stop eating. Humans have the unfortunate ability to override this feeling. For example, you can eat ice cream if you so desire even after you have finished eating a large meal. You can eat when you wish, not just when your body requires nourishment. You should learn to control this ability to override nutritional needs by learning to recognize those internal signals that the body produces in response to a true need for food. To do so, you must learn to distinguish between true hunger and the desire to keep on eating, and then eat *only* when you are hungry and *only* the amount needed to satisfy your feelings of hunger, *not* the amount of food you feel you enjoy eating.

Scientific knowledge about what causes the feeling of satiation is less advanced than the knowledge about hunger—and knowledge about hunger is still in its infancy! When science develops a better understanding of what produces the sensation of satiation, it will be possible to develop ways to produce this response without overeating, thereby preventing obesity as a result of overeating. Happily, this potential is not as distant as one might fear.

Heredity vs. Conditioned Response

Is being fat a hereditary state? When we look at over-weight fathers and sons or mothers and daughters who are identical in size and shape, it seems likely. In fact, examples of this kind of obesity can be found in three generations in families, leading one to believe that heredity causes it. Studies have shown that in families where both parents are of normal weight, only 9 percent of the children are obese. On the other hand, when one parent is overweight, 40 percent of the children are obese, and when both parents are over-weight, 80 percent of the children are obese.

It is hard to say whether this is the result of heredity or whether parents who eat too much educate their children to overeat, whereas thin parents set an example for their children, who also stay thin. Certainly the kinds of diets that children are raised on and learn to like have something to do with their ultimate body structure.

Learned Habits

The concept of "learned" eating habits was heightened for me by a recent incident in my office. I was seeing a couple who had been married for a year. The wife, who was five feet, six inches tall and weighed 190 pounds, was having some medical problems; I suggested that she reduce her weight. The weight loss would help correct her specific problems, and it would be a good general-health measure. She replied that it was extremely difficult for her to lose weight because her husband brought home ice cream every night and encouraged her to eat it with him.

He agreed, saying, "I can't help it. I love ice cream and I was unable to have it when I was young, so I really enjoy eating it now."

She shook her head and said to me: "I tell him that he will have to stop or else I'll get to weigh a ton."

She's right, if not in the literal sense. She will weigh a ton in terms of the damage to her health. Unless she controls her caloric intake, she will be in serious trouble before too long.

Consider that this couple is trying to have a child. Unless something changes, the child will be part of a home of overeaters. The child will be educated to eat. Heredity will be a secondary consideration. If the child is obese, it will result from learned attitudes toward food and eating.

Overfeeding Your Children Can Have Lifetime Consequences

There are other reasons why overfeeding a child is believed to play an important role in developing an obese adult. Early in childhood your food intake determines the number of fat cells you will have in your body for the remainder of your life. If you are overfed, your body will develop a large number of fat cells. If you are fed only the required volume of food, your body will produce only the number of fat cells needed for your size. The presence of an abnormally large number of fat cells results in obesity; the result is a conditioned response rather than a hereditary factor.

You may have gotten off to the wrong start as a child, but that's no excuse for now—and it isn't too late to make adjustments in your *present* eating habits. Eating less is a small price to pay for lowered blood pressure and better general health.

7 ~~~

Eat Right to Feel Right

Assuming you have decided the time has come to reduce, what should you do next? The simplest step is to reduce your food intake by half. This may sound difficult, but it's effective. Also, the reduction makes the change to a nutritionally sound diet less difficult. Count your calories. Keep a record as you progress. This written record will help you replace certain foods with others that have a lower caloric value. If you are accustomed to eating two slices of bread at lunch, cut down to one slice. Next, try to replace this one slice with something that is more filling and has fewer calories.

Dieting becomes simple once you develop the necessary self-control. You need not even ask what you should eat and what you should avoid. Today most people know exactly what is high in calories and what is not. It is common knowledge that candy, ice cream, potato chips, beer, cake, and sugar in all its forms should be avoided. To stay away from these high-calo-

Calorie Content of Common Foods

Food Item	Common Measure (Weight, g)	Calories
Beverages (Alcoholic)		
Beer, regular	12-oz can or bottle (360)	151
Beer, light	12-oz can or bottle (360)	70–136
Brandy	1½ fl oz (45)	105
Gin (86 proof)	1½ fl oz (45)	105
Rum (86 proof)	1½ fl oz (45)	105
Vodka (86 proof)	1½ fl oz (45)	105
Whiskey, bourbon, rye, or scotch (86 proof)	1½ fl oz (45)	105
Wine, red domestic	4 fl oz (120)	99
Wine, red imported	4 fl oz (120)	99
Wine, sherry	4 fl oz (120)	151
Wine, white domestic	4 fl oz (120)	99
Wine, white imported	4 fl oz (120)	99
Beverages (Nonalcoholic)		
Apple juice	6 fl oz (180)	87
Coffee, brewed	1 cup—8 fl oz (240)	0
Coffee, instant	1 cup—8 fl oz (240)	2
Cranberry juice cocktail	6 fl oz (180)	123
Grape juice, bottled or canned	6 fl oz (190)	125
Orange juice, fresh	6 fl oz (180)	84
Orange juice, frozen	6 fl oz (186)	92
Pineapple juice	6 fl oz (188)	69
Prune juice	6 fl oz (192	149
Soft drinks		
Regular	8 fl oz (240)	96
Diet	8 fl oz (240)	1
Club soda	8 fl oz (240)	0
Collins mix	8 fl oz (240)	112
Quinine water (tonic)	8 fl oz (240)	72
Mineral water	8 fl oz (240)	0
Tomato juice	6 fl oz (192)	36
Tea	1 cup—8 fl oz (240)	0
Tea, instant	1 cup—8 fl oz (240)	0
Vegetable juice cocktail	6 fl oz (182)	30
Breads and Crackers		
Biscuit, home recipe	1 biscuit (28)	103
Biscuit, mix, with milk	1 biscuit (28)	104
Bread, French	1 slice (23)	64
Bread, pumpernickel	1 slice (32)	79
Bread, rye	1 slice (25)	61

Calorie Content of Common Foods (continued)

Food Item	Common Measure (Weight, g)	Calories
Bread, white	1 slice (25)	76
Bread, whole wheat	1 slice (25)	61
Bread stick, salt coating	1 stick, small (10)	38
Bread stick, without salt coating	1 stick, small (10)	38
Cracker, saltine or soda	1 cracker (3)	12
Cracker, soup or oyster	10 crackers (8)	33
Roll, dinner, brown and serve	1 roll (28)	83
Roll, frankfurter, hamburger	1 roll (40)	119
Roll, hard	1 roll (50)	156

Cereals (Non-Sugar-Coated)

Food Item	Common Measure (Weight, g)	Calories
Bran, all	1 oz—⅓ cup (28)	70
Bran flakes (40%)	1 oz—⅔ cup (28)	90
Corn flakes	1 oz—1 cup (28)	110
Corn Chex	1 oz—1 cup (28)	110
Granola	1 oz—¼ cup (28)	130
Grits, cooked	1 oz—¾ cup (28)	100
Oat flakes	1 oz—⅔ cup (28)	100
Oatmeal, regular, without salt	1 oz—⅓ cup (28)	109
Oatmeal, instant, regular flavor (salt added)	1 oz—¾ cup (28)	105
Rice, Cream of, unsalted	1 oz—¾ cup (28)	110
Rice, puffed	½ oz—1 heaping cup (14)	50
Rice Chex	1 oz—1⅛ cup (28)	110
Rice Krispies	1 oz—1 cup (28)	110
Wheat Chex	1 oz—⅔ cup (28)	110
Wheat, Cream of, regular	1 oz—¾ cup (28)	110
Wheat flakes	1 oz—1 cup (28)	110
Wheat, puffed	½ oz—1 heaping cup (14)	50
Wheat, shredded	1 large biscuit (21)	80

Condiments, Dressings, and Seasonings

Food Item	Common Measure (Weight, g)	Calories
Barbecue sauce	1 tbsp (16)	14
Catsup, tomato	1 tbsp (15)	16
Chili sauce	1 tbsp (17)	16
Mayonnaise	1 tbsp (15)	101
Mustard, prepared	1 tsp (5)	5
Parsley flakes	1 tbsp (4)	2
Pepper, black	1 tsp (2)	8
Salad dressings		
Bleu cheese or Roquefort	1 tbsp (15)	76
French	1 tbsp (14)	66
Italian	1 tbsp (15)	83

Calorie Content of Common Foods (continued)

Food Item	Common Measure (Weight, g)	Calories
Russian	1 tbsp (15)	74
Thousand Island	1 tbsp (16)	80
Oil and vinegar	1 tbsp (15)	62
Salt, table	1 tsp (6)	0
Soy sauce	1 tbsp (18)	12
Sugar, granulated	1 tsp (4)	15
Worcestershire sauce	1 tbsp (17)	Trace

Dairy Products, Eggs, and Margarine

Food Item	Common Measure (Weight, g)	Calories
Butter, regular	1 tbsp (14)	102
Butter, whipped	1 tbsp (9)	69
Butter, unsalted, regular	1 tbsp (14)	102
Cheese, American	1 slice—1 oz (28)	116
Cheese, cheddar	1 oz (28)	114
Cheese, cottage	½ cup (113)	117
Cheese, cream	1 oz (28)	99
Cheese, Parmesan, grated	1 oz (28)	129
Cheese, Swiss	1 oz (28)	107
Cheese, processed spread	1 oz (28)	82
Cream, half and half	1 tbsp (15)	20
Cream, heavy	1 tbsp (15)	53
Cream, sour	1 tbsp (12)	26
Egg, whole	1 medium (50)	79
Egg, white	1 medium (33)	16
Egg, yolk	1 medium (17)	63
Margarine, regular	1 tbsp (14)	100
Margarine, soft, tub	1 tbsp (14)	100
Margarine, unsalted	1 tbsp (14)	100
Milk, buttermilk	8 fl oz (245)	99
Milk, low-fat (2%)	8 fl oz (244)	121
Milk, skim	8 fl oz (245)	86
Milk, whole	8 fl oz (244)	150

Desserts

Food Item	Common Measure (Weight, g)	Calories
Brownies	1 average (20)	97
Cake, angel food	1 slice, ½2 cake (56)	150
Cake, devil's food, chocolate icing	1 slice, ½2 cake (67)	260
Cake, pound	1 medium slice (55)	225
Cake, white, white icing	1 slice, ½2 cake (104)	290
Cake, yellow, with caramel icing	1 slice, ½2 cake (108)	391
Cookies, chocolate chip	1 cookie, medium (11)	50

Calorie Content of Common Foods (continued)

Food Item	Common Measure (Weight, g)	Calories
Cookies, sandwich	1 cookie (10)	63
Cookies, oatmeal	1 cookie (13)	120
Cookies, sugar	1 cookie (26)	128
Cookies, fig	1 bar (14)	56
Cookies, vanilla wafer	1 wafer (4)	16
Cookies, shortbread	1 cookie (8)	37
Gelatin, plain	½ cup (120)	80
Ice cream	1 cup (140)	257
Ice milk	1 cup (131)	199
Pie, apple	1 slice, ⅛ pie (71)	182
Pie, banana cream	1 slice, ⅛ pie (66)	126
Pie, blueberry	1 slice, ⅛ pie (71)	172
Pie, cherry	1 slice, ⅛ pie (71)	185
Pie, chocolate cream	1 slice, ⅛ pie (66)	174
Pie, lemon meringue	1 slice, ⅛ pie (105)	268
Pie, mince	1 slice, ⅛ pie (71)	259
Pie, peach	1 slice, ⅛ pie (71)	150
Pie, pecan	1 slice, ⅛ pie (71)	259
Pie, pumpkin	1 slice, ⅛ pie (71)	150
Pudding, bread	½ cup (133)	248
Pudding, chocolate, home recipe	½ cup (130)	198
Pudding, chocolate, mix	½ cup (148)	322
Pudding, rice	½ cup (132)	194
Pudding, tapioca	½ cup (83)	111
Pudding, vanilla, home recipe	½ cup (128)	142
Pudding, vanilla, mix	½ cup (148)	321
Sherbet, orange	1 cup (193)	259

Fish and Seafood

Food Item	Common Measure (Weight, g)	Calories
Bluefish, broiled or baked with butter	4 oz (114)	219
Clams, raw	4 to 5—3 oz (85)	56
Cod, broiled with butter	4 oz (114)	99
Crabmeat, canned, drained	1 can—4 oz (114)	126
Flounder, baked with butter	4 oz (114)	102
Haddock, fried	4 oz (114)	162
Halibut, broiled with butter	4 oz (114)	191
Lobster, boiled, meat only	4 oz (114)	123
Oysters, fresh	6 small—2 oz (58)	38
Salmon, broiled or baked with butter	4 oz (114)	207

Calorie Content of Common Foods (continued)

Food Item	Common Measure (Weight, g)	Calories
Sardines, drained	1 can—3¼ oz (92)	187
Scallops, bay, steamed	10 to 12—4 oz (114)	153
Shrimp, raw	10 jumbo—3 oz (85)	98
Tuna, chunk, canned in oil, drained	1 can—3¼ oz (92)	182
Tuna, chunk, canned in water, drained	1 can—3¼ oz (92)	117

Fruits

Apple	1 medium (138)	118
Applesauce, sweetened	½ cup (125)	227
Apricots, canned, syrup	½ cup (129)	111
Apricots, dried	5 halves, medium (24)	62
Banana	1 medium (119)	68
Blackberries	½ cup (72)	42
Blueberries	½ cup (72)	45
Cantaloupe	½ melon (272)	47
Cherries, sweet, whole	1 cup (130)	82
Cherries, canned	1 cup (257)	110
Fruit cocktail, canned in syrup	1 cup (255)	195
Fruit cocktail, canned in water	1 cup (255)	95
Grapefruit	½ grapefruit (120)	26
Grapefruit, canned	½ cup (127)	89
Grapes	10 grapes (50)	23
Honeydew	⅙ melon (298)	61
Orange	1 medium (131)	47
Peach, skinned	1 medium (100)	29
Peach, canned, syrup	½ cup (128)	100
Peaches, canned, water	½ cup (128)	38
Pear	1 medium (168)	93
Pears, canned, syrup	½ cup (128)	98
Pears, canned, water	½ cup (128)	40
Pineapple, fresh	1 cup (135)	71
Pineapple, canned, syrup	1 cup (265)	169
Pineapple, canned, water	1 cup (246)	96
Plums	10 plums (66)	30
Plums, canned, water	1 cup (256)	111
Prunes, cooked	½ cup (107)	108
Prunes, dried	5 prunes (43)	95
Raisins	¼ cup, packed (36)	98
Rhubarb, cooked, sweetened	½ cup (135)	190
Strawberries	½ cup (75)	28

Calorie Content of Common Foods (continued)

Food Item	Common Measure (Weight, g)	Calories
Strawberries, frozen, sweetened ½ cup (128)		139
Watermelon	1/16 melon (426)	65

Meat and Poultry

Food Item	Common Measure (Weight, g)	Calories
Bacon, regular	2 slices—½ oz (14)	61
Bacon, Canadian	1 slice—1 oz (28)	58
Bologna	1 slice (22)	61
Beef, corned	2 slices—3 oz (80)	315
Beef, dried, creamed	1 cup (245)	377
Beef, ground, lean	1 patty—4 oz (114)	249
Beef, lean, rump roast	2 slices—4 oz (114)	237
Beef, lean, round steak	6 oz (170)	444
Chicken, broiler	¼ chicken (147)	120
Chicken, roasted	½ breast (98)	99
Chicken, fried	1 drumstick (56)	68
Frankfurter, all meat	1 frankfurter (57)	176
Ham, cured, lean	2 slices—4 oz (114)	330
Ham, cured, country, lean	2 slices—4 oz (144)	304
Ham, fresh, lean	2 slices—4 oz (114)	426
Ham, chopped lunchmeat	1 slice (21)	62
Ham, deviled	1 oz (28)	100
Lamb, loin chop, lean	2 chops—4 oz (114)	214
Lamb, leg, lean	2 slices—4 oz (114)	212
Liver, calf, fried	3 slices—4 oz (114)	298
Liver, chicken, simmered	5 livers—4 oz (114)	188
Liverwurst (braunschweiger)	1 slice (28)	88
Pork, loin roast, lean	1 slice—4 oz (114)	292
Salami, dry, beef and pork	1 slice (10)	45
Salami, cooked, beef and pork	1 slice (22)	88
Sausage, pork	1 link (13)	65
Sausage, pork	1 patty—2 oz (57)	129
Thuringer (summer sausage)	1 slice (22)	68
Turkey, dark meat	3 slices—4 oz (114)	218
Turkey, light meat	3 slices—4 oz (114)	200
Turkey, roll	1 oz (28)	70
Veal, cutlet, loin	1 cutlet—4 oz (114)	267

Pasta

Food Item	Common Measure (Weight, g)	Calories
Macaroni, plain, cooked	1 cup (140)	155
Macaroni with cheese	1 cup (200)	430
Pizza with cheese	1 slice—2 oz (57)	147
Pizza with sausage	1 slice—2 oz (57)	157

Calorie Content of Common Foods (continued)

Food Item	Common Measure (Weight, g)	Calories
Spaghetti, with tomato sauce and cheese	1 cup (250)	190
Spaghetti, with tomato sauce, meatballs, and cheese	1 cup (248)	332

Soups, Commercial Varieties, Condensed (Prepared with Addition of Equal Volumes of Water, Unless Noted)

Bean	1 cup (250)	168
Beef broth	1 cup (241)	64
Chicken, cream of (with milk)	1 cup (245)	179
Chicken noodle	1 cup (240)	62
Chicken with rice	1 cup (241)	48
Clam chowder, Manhattan	1 cup (244)	81
Clam chowder, New England (with milk)	1 cup (248)	139
Minestrone	1 cup (241)	105
Mushroom, cream of (with milk)	1 cup (248)	216
Onion	1 cup (240)	65
Pea, green	1 cup (250)	130
Tomato	1 cup (245)	88
Tomato, cream of (with milk)	1 cup (250)	173
Turkey noodle	1 cup (240)	79
Vegetable beef	1 cup (245)	78
Vegetarian vegetable	1 cup (245)	78

Vegetables (Considered Fresh, Unless Listed Otherwise; Considered Cooked, Unless Indicated as Raw)

Artichoke	1 bud (120)	12
Asparagus	4 spears (60)	12
Asparagus, canned	4 spears (80)	17
Beans, baked, canned with pork and tomato sauce	½ cup (145)	156
Beans, baked, canned, with pork and molasses sauce	½ cup (145)	192
Beans, green	½ cup (63)	16
Beans, green, canned	½ cup (65)	16
Beans, green, frozen	½ cup (68)	17
Beans, lima	½ cup (85)	95
Beans, lima, canned	½ cup (85)	82
Beans, lima, frozen	½ cup (85)	84
Beets	½ cup (85)	27

Calorie Content of Common Foods (continued)

Food Item	Common Measure (Weight, g)	Calories
Beets, canned	½ cup (85)	42
Broccoli	1 stalk, medium (151)	39
Broccoli, frozen	½ cup (94)	24
Brussels sprouts	4 sprouts (84)	30
Brussels sprouts, frozen	½ cup (77)	26
Cabbage	½ cup (72)	16
Cabbage, raw	½ cup (35)	11
Carrots	½ cup (78)	34
Carrots, frozen	½ cup (113)	35
Carrots, raw	1 medium (72)	12
Cauliflower	½ cup (63)	14
Cauliflower, frozen	½ cup (90)	16
Cauliflower, raw	½ cup (58)	14
Celery, raw	1 stalk (20)	7
Corn	1 ear (140)	70
Corn, canned, creamed	½ cup (128)	105
Corn, canned, whole kernel	½ cup (83)	87
Cucumber, raw	6 large slices (28)	4
Lettuce, head, raw	¼ head (135)	18
Lettuce, leaf, raw	1 cup (55)	10
Mushrooms	½ cup (35)	10
Okra	5 pods (53)	16
Onions, green, raw, with tops	2 medium (30)	14
Onions, raw	1 tbsp (10)	4
Peas, green	½ cup (80)	57
Peas, green, canned	½ cup (85)	82
Peas, green, frozen	½ cup (85)	55
Peppers, sweet	½ cup (75)	22
Pickles, dill	1 spear (30)	3
Pickles, sweet gherkin	1 whole pickle (15)	22
Potato, baked or boiled	1 medium (158)	145
Potatoes, french fried, unsalted	10 strips (50)	137
Potatoes, mashed, milk and salt added	1 cup (210)	137
Radishes, raw	5 medium (18)	7
Sauerkraut	½ cup (235)	21
Spinach, canned	½ cup (103)	25
Spinach, frozen	½ cup (50)	24
Spinach, raw	½ cup (55)	7
Squash, summer	½ cup (105)	13
Sweet potato, boiled	1 medium (132)	126
Sweet potato, canned	1 medium (100)	107

Calorie Content of Common Foods (continued)		
Food Item	Common Measure (Weight, g)	Calories
Tomato, raw	1 medium (123)	27
Tomatoes, canned	½ cup (120)	26
Snacks		
Caramels, plain or chocolate	1 oz (28)	113
Candy, milk chocolate	1 oz (28)	147
Corn chips, regular	1 oz (28)	157
Doughnuts, cake type, plain	1 doughnut (32)	125
Mints, chocolate-coated	1 small (11)	45
Nuts, cashews, dry-roasted, salted	4 tbsp—1 oz (28)	159
Peanut butter	1 tbsp—1 oz (16)	94
Peanuts, dry-roasted, salted	4 tbsp—1 oz (28)	166
Peanuts, roasted in oil, unsalted	4 tbsp—1 oz (28)	206
Popcorn, salted, with butter	1 cup (9)	41
Popcorn, unsalted	1 cup (6)	23
Potato chips	14 chips—1 oz (26)	161
Pretzels, regular twist	5 pretzels—½ oz. (14)	117

rie items, replace them with more calorie-intelligent items, such as fruits, vegetables, and grains. (The table on pages 72–80 gives calorie counts for many of the foods we eat.)

Just How Many Calories Do You Need?

How much food you should consume depends, obviously, on your size and your activities. Of course, this figure will vary, depending on age and sex. As a rule, males eighteen years and over need 2,400 to 3,000 calories per day; females eighteen and over need 1,800 to 2,100 calories daily.

Weight-reduction diets can range from 900 to 1,800 calories per day. The basic concept is that each day you should take in about 500 fewer calories than your body normally needs for maintenance. This sort of diet should produce a weight loss of between one and two pounds a week—the right amount, since a slow, constant loss is better than a rapid one. A slow diet allows your body to adjust to the new level of calories. Once you have lost the weight you wanted to lose, you must try to maintain it by watching your intake of calories.

I think diets like the Pritikin that start at an uncomfortably low calorie level make it too hard for most dieters. On the basis of my experience as well as for practical reasons, I recommend two dietary levels: the first, for weight reduction, is a 1,200-calorie diet; the second, for maintenance, is a 2,000-calorie diet. If you start at too low a level you tend not to maintain that level no matter how good your original intentions might be. By starting at a more reasonable level of 1,200 calories, you are more likely to accomplish your goal. A 2,000-calorie maintenance diet is also generally at the right level. If you find it is too high or too low, you can adjust it once you become accustomed to eating the right foods in the right proportions.

If You Are Eating More Than You Should

Now that you know how many calories you need each day, I'd like to add some things you can do when trying to eliminate calorie-rich foods from your life:

- Don't go shopping for food when you are hungry. I have made careful note of the shopping I have done after lunch as opposed to the shopping I have done before supper, when I am hungry. When you are hungry you buy many items you would not consider if you were satisfied. I noted an increase in the appeal of cake and bread when I shopped before meals rather than after meals. The safe way to shop is to make a list of those items you need and include on that list only the things that meet your diet plan. Do not buy items on impulse. Just because peach ice cream is on sale does not mean you must buy the gallon size and indulge yourself. Stay with your predetermined diet plan. Have a list and adhere to it. Buy nothing more.

- Prepare in advance for the TV hunger rush— that sudden craving to eat something when you are watching television. Keep celery sticks, carrots, pineapple pieces, sunflower seeds, raisins, low-calorie soda, and no-salt, no-butter popcorn on hand, or make a bailout emergency list of your own to meet this problem.

- Do not keep calorie-rich snack food at home. I find that if there are cookies or cakes that I like easily available in the kitchen, the temptation to walk in and take them is too great. If these foods are not available I will happily eat an apple, a banana, or other fruit as a substitute. As a matter of fact, I have gotten so accustomed to these replacements that I find I no longer enjoy candy as I did in the past—it tastes too sweet!

- A food scale is an invaluable aid in controlling your food intake. There are many foods that are acceptable if you simply limit the amount you eat. If you can safely have three ounces of an item, you can use the scale to measure the weight exactly. Many things can be eaten in small amounts, even though they are high in calories. Learn to limit the amount, and weigh it to be sure.

- Keep an accurate record of all you eat. In reviewing your daily intake of food, it sometimes comes as a shock to discover how much more you are eating than you thought.

- Weigh yourself each day, and keep a careful record of your successes and failures while dieting. If you start to go up in weight, reduce your intake the next day to help balance the increase. Even if you do well dieting, there will be times when you go off for one reason or another. Do not allow this slight deviation to be the end of your diet. On the contrary, use the deviation to help you get back to dieting with greater resolution. The next day just balance out the excess intake you had the day before by eating less. Use the scale to measure how well you are doing. After a while you won't even need the scale—just looking in the mirror will tell all.

- As soon as you have lost some weight and maintained the loss for a week or so, have your clothing altered to fit. The smaller size is a great incentive to encourage you to stay at your new weight. As soon as the clothing starts to get a little tight you know you should get down to some serious dieting again.

- Many people find that changing the way they chew food can help. If you try to chew food slowly, you may find you will feel more satisfied with less. Allow some time to pass between taking a bite and chewing it. You can increase your sense of satiation with less food simply by spending more time eating. Try this yourself—it is easy to do and well worth the effort. Indeed, there may be a relationship between the time spent eating and/or sitting at the table and the amount of food needed to feel satisfied. Thin people tend to sit at the table for longer periods and pick at food, whereas the overweight eat large amounts at a faster rate.

Diet and Exercise

Everybody has always told you that exercise helps lose those pounds. And everybody was right. However, you have to exercise a *lot* to make up for indulging in fattening foods. Here are explanations of how much exercise you need to remove the calories in (a) a glass of wine, (b) a fried egg, and (c) a soda.

To burn off one 3½-ounce glass of dry white wine (85 calories) requires:

- 6 minutes of running 7.5 miles per hour for a loss of 13.2 calories per minute
- 22 minutes of walking 3 miles per hour for a loss of 3.8 calories per minute
- 10 minutes of swimming for a loss of 8.1 calories per minute

To burn off one fried egg (115 calories) requires:

- 9 minutes of running
- 30 minutes of walking
- 14 minutes of swimming

To burn off one cola soda (145 calories) requires:

- 11 minutes of running
- 38 minutes of walking
- 18 minutes of swimming

Since your weight is a balance between the calories you take in and those you use up, you can now work both ends against the middle. You can increase your exercise as you cut your calories; it's just like burning the candle at both ends, only better for you.

Begin by determining how many calories you are taking in daily. Next, study the following examples to get an idea of the number of calories used up in various forms of exercise.

Activity	*Calories*
Walking up stairs	20 per minute
Running (at rate of 7 mph)	12–14 per minute
Running/jogging (moderate rate)	10–12 per minute
Bicycling (at rate of 13 mph)	10–12 per minute
Walking (at rate of 4.5 mph)	6–7 per minute
Walking (at rate of 3 mph)	50–100 per mile
Skating (moderately vigorously)	5–7 per minute
Handball	9–10 per minute
Swimming (rapidly)	9–11 per minute
Tennis (strong game)	9–10 per minute
Cross-country skiing (at rate of 5 mph)	11–12 per minute
Downhill skiing (light turns)	8–10 per minute

Folk dancing/disco dancing	6–9 per minute
Rowing	7–8 per minute

Now determine how many calories you are burning up by exercising. Fill in the following chart for one week; estimate your caloric expenditure by using the preceding table.

You will very quickly be able to see the relationship between what you are taking in and how much you are working off—and it won't be hard to understand why; if you are sedentary and have a big appetite, you just keep putting on weight. Once you really understand how much exercise you need to burn up just a few calories, you may come to the conclusion that one of the best exercises is pushing away from the table.

While exercise is beneficial to your general health and is of particular help in lowering blood pressure, it is not the perfect route to weight loss.

What Else You Can Do

1. *Watch your intake of salt.* Because salt causes the body to retain fluid, adding to weight, avoid or cut down on the following:

   dill pickles
   salted butter or margarine
   onion, garlic, or celery salts
   olives
   salted and smoked fish
   canned tomatoes as well as many other canned vegetables

Any of the following foods are recommended (used within your caloric needs):

broccoli	lettuce	cucumbers
green and red	radishes	mushrooms
peppers	chicken	spinach
zucchini	skim milk	fish
veal	bananas	apples
oranges	cantaloupes	grapes
raisins	strawberries	grapefruit
prunes	pasta	whole-grain
coffee	seltzer	unsweetened
tea	low-calorie,	cereals
celery	low-salt soda	unsalted
		nuts

2. *Increase your carbohydrate consumption* so it accounts for 55 to 60 percent of calorie (energy) intake.

   Carbohydrates are the starches and sugars that occur in fruits and vegetables and in pastries, breads, and anything that has sugar or flour as its base. Starches and simple sugars such as glucose supply about 50 percent of the body's energy needs and should be increased to 55 to 60 percent for optimum health. The foods that help supply carbohydrates include:

   - rice
   - potatoes
   - spaghetti
   - bread
   - cereal
   - certain fruits such as bananas, oranges, all kinds of dried beans (lentils, lima beans, kidney beans, etc.), corn, sweet potatoes, and yams

   Remember that you must still keep track of the number of calories you are taking in, or you may find that the increase in sugar will cause you to become obese. As a nation, we tend to be sugar junkies; we eat everything sugar-coated or "sugar added." Try to reduce the intake of pure sugar by removing the sugar bowl from the table and avoiding sugar-filled soft drinks. Avoid eating foods that have a high sugar content, and read labels so you can avoid dextrose, corn syrup, and sucrose, because they all mean sugar. Don't be fooled by honey: It is really sugar in disguise. And don't assume that "all natural" means "no sugar." It doesn't.

3. *Reduce the total consumption of fat* from approximately 40 percent to 30 percent.

Our diets contain too much fat, and while fat gives food flavor and an appealing juiciness, we should decrease its consumption. Too much fat increases the danger of arteriosclerosis by allowing the buildup of fat deposits in the blood vessels. A high-fat diet not only makes you fat, it also increases the risk of cancer of the colon, breast, and prostate. Unfortunately, there is no substitute for fat; you simply must cut out foods that have a high fat content, such as red meats (particularly beef and pork), butter, lard, unsweetened chocolate (which is about 50 percent fat), nuts, peanut butter, bacon, luncheon meats, frankfurters, and doughnuts.

4. *Reduce the consumption of saturated fats*, which should account for only 10 percent of the daily dietary intake, and substitute polyunsaturated and monounsaturated fats.

Saturated fats are solid at room temperature and are found mainly in meat and in dairy products such as butter, milk, and cheese. *Unsaturated fats*, which are liquid at room temperature, are obtained from plants and include safflower oil, corn oil, peanut oil, and soybean and cottonseed oils.

5. *Reduce the consumption of cholesterol* to about 300 mg a day.
   Limit or eliminate:

- eggs
- most cheeses
- organ meats
- fats
- butter
- bacon
- beef
- coconut oil
- palm oil

Whenever possible, substitute polyunsaturated fats such as:

- corn oil
- safflower oil
- soybean and sesame oils
- fish oils

Other Techniques When All Else Fails

- *Behavior modification* is a concept based on Pavlov's experiments (in which he conditioned a dog to salivate on hearing a bell because the dog had been trained to know that a bell sounded when he was to be fed). In dietary behavior modification, food is associated with an electric shock or some other type of unpleasant

	Exercise	Length of Time	Estimated Value in Calories
Monday			
Tuesday			
Wednesday			
Thursday			
Friday			
Saturday			
Sunday			

phenomenon. People who have stayed with this type of therapy have found it successful. However, it is time-consuming and unpleasant, and for that reason most drop out.

- *The carrot-on-a-stick approach* also can be applied to dieting. I have two friends, physicians and partners, who have agreed to pay each other a dollar reward for each pound of weight lost. Unfortunately, so far this has not worked too well, and neither has lost much weight. I believe the problem here is that motivation is basic to weight loss and that this type of external encouragement is insufficient.

- *Psychotherapy*, both in groups and individually, has been tried with some success, as has hypnosis, but results have not been impressive.

In abnormally obese people, *surgery* to shorten the intestinal tract so that the passageway absorbs less food has been tried. This is *not* a satisfactory option and should not be considered.

Don't Forget Your Nutritional Needs

It's easy to lose sight of your body's nutritional requirements while your mind is focused on weight loss. When choosing "thin" foods that help you diet, don't forget about energy requirements, body type, age, and overall good health as well as special conditions, such as pregnancy. The caloric needs and therefore the effects of a decreased caloric intake are quite different in a six-foot-four male weighing 250 pounds than in a five-foot-six male of the same weight. The shorter man will lose more weight on a low-calorie diet than will the taller, but the diets would have to be adjusted to their respective sizes, and the optimum weight for each would differ: A weight of 207 pounds would be the maximum desirable for the six-foot-four male, whereas 164 pounds would be right for the five-foot-six male.

Each person is so different from every other person that a method that works for one will not necessarily work for another. Some people lose weight more easily than others. However, there are some basic guidelines that will enable you to keep your weight down and still remain healthy.

The Ten Nutrition Commandments

Following are ten commandments that, if followed, will lead to good nutritional health:

Thou shalt not eat an unbalanced or unvaried diet.

Thou shalt not disregard your calorie count—keep it sacred.

Thou shalt change your eating habits.

Thou shalt listen to your internal body signals and eat *only* when you feel hungry.

Thou shalt not eat because of social, emotional, or enticement pressures.

Thou shalt not eat incorrect foods, only correct ones.

Thou shalt not eat too much salt or sugar.

Thou shalt not eat too much cholesterol or saturated fat.

Thou shalt not drink too much alcohol.

Thou shalt increase the number of fiber foods you eat.

8 ≋

The Rice Diet

The major advance in our understanding of the relationship between diet and the treatment of hypertension was made by Dr. Walter Kempner of Duke University, who was responsible for what has come to be known as "the rice diet."

In the early 1940s Kempner began treating patients with kidney disease with a low-protein diet on the theory that a low-protein diet would put less work load on the kidneys and thus give them a chance to heal, an idea that still has many supporters.

The Rice Diet's Effect on Hypertension

Kempner's subsequent discovery that there was a relationship between the rice diet and the control of hypertension was purely fortuitous. Kempner had placed a thirty-three-year-old woman suffering from severe kidney disease on the rice diet. He told her to remain on the diet for two weeks and then come back for further evaluation. She misunderstood Kempner's instructions, however, and returned to see him after she had been on the diet for two months. When he reexamined her, Kempner found a remarkable change in her physical condition: Her blood pressure had come down, and her electrocardiogram had improved, as had the serious aspects of her kidney disease. Seeing this marked change, Kempner quickly realized that long-term dietary treatment must be the answer; the short-term diet was too brief to produce these results.

After the First Case, Five Hundred More

Kempner studied five hundred patients before reporting his findings on the success of this diet to the medical community. He found that in almost two-thirds of his patients, blood pressure decreased, kidney function improved, and cardiac muscle was strengthened as evidenced by improvement in the electrocardiogram.

Thereafter, many people with kidney disease were placed on this diet, staying in what came to be known as the Rice Houses of Duke University. Once the use of the rice diet was instituted in hypertensive patients, it became clear that it produced a marked improvement in blood pressure, and Kempner's work began to be accepted widely. This marked the beginning of the use of low-salt diets to treat patients with high blood pressure, the only method that was successful in the era before the advent of the present-day antihypertensive medications. Even today, low-salt diets continue to hold an important place in the treatment of patients with high blood pressure.

What made the rice diet so effective? Kempner felt it was a combination of the rigid restriction of protein and fat coupled with a decrease in both sodium and chloride intake. Not everyone was to agree with this conclusion. In 1945, Drs. A. Grollman and T. R. Harrison reported in the *Journal of the American Medical Association* that patients could be treated successfully without such a severe regimen of protein restriction as long as the sodium intake was kept down.

Drawbacks to the Rice Diet

Given Kempner's success, what prevented the widespread use of this diet? If it was so very good, why wasn't everyone with high blood pressure, kidney disease, or obesity put on it?

Unfortunately, the rice diet is both difficult to administer and extremely difficult to follow consistently. The present rice diet at Duke University consists of rice, fruit, and no salt, with between twenty-four and forty ounces of liquid daily. As such, it has twice as much carbohydrate as the average American diet, one-fourth as much protein, and less than one-twentieth the amount of fat. The diet is, of course, adjusted to the individual's special needs. However, one consistent hurdle is the monotony of the diet. Large volumes of rice eaten daily are not very exciting fare.

Patients who are on the diet at Duke University must be monitored regularly to make sure that they remain on the diet. This is done by collecting a twenty-four-hour urine specimen each week and analyzing its chemical content. Since the chemical constituents of urine change with diet, it is possible to spot any transgressions quickly.

Another problem with the rice diet is that it requires three to five days of preliminary diagnostic studies before a person starts the program. It also involves months of treatment, and during this time patients must find living quarters while they are taking the special meals. All of this is expensive and assumes that one has blocks of time available. The doctors at Duke say that you can diet with this method at home but that you need the group support and the medical support you can only obtain at Duke. Their experiences are probably correct. The rice diet is a difficult one to do on your own.

However, when you weigh all these drawbacks against such complications of high blood pressure as stroke, heart attack, heart failure, and hypertension-induced sexual impotence in the male, the diet may not be so hard to accept after all.

The diet is not for all hypertensives. Some people with a certain type of kidney disease do not do well with too restrictive a reduction of salt. While this is not a common problem, it constitutes yet another drawback to this treatment.

Why Rice?

When Dr. Kempner chose rice as the staple of the diet, was it another purely fortuitous decision, or was there something about rice that made him select it?

It would seem it was a thought-out decision. As a food, rice offers all the qualities needed for this type of dietary restriction. It is free of salt and cholesterol, low in calories, high in bulk, and easy to prepare.

Rice is not a newcomer to the pages of medical history. In fact, it holds an interesting place in the development of the relationship between diet and disease. As far back as 1897, a Dutch physician named Eijkman, working in a prison hospital in Java, noted that poultry fed on polished rice developed a disease of the nervous system similar to beriberi in man. When chickens were fed the part of the rice that had been removed in the process of polishing, the symptoms of the disease abated. The missing essential ingredient was found to be vitamin B_1, or thiamine, which is retained when rice is not processed by polishing.

Thus the nutritive value of rice varies, depending on whether or not it is milled or polished or parboiled. In the natural state, rice, which is really a grass, has a coarse outside, or hull. When this hull is removed, the grain of rice is still brown because it has a covering of bran, which contains all the vitamins and minerals. Brown rice is rice with this bran coating intact; when rice is milled or polished, it becomes white and simultaneously loses much of its vitamin nutritional value, especially B_1 vitamin. In Asia, four types of rice are eaten. The Asian white is as poor nutritionally as ours. People in the Philippines eat yellow rice, brown rice, and red rice. Each has different nutritional values. Since most Americans prefer white rice, methods have been developed whereby rice can be parboiled—or converted—before milling to preserve some of its nutritional value. In this process, the unmilled rice is soaked in water just under the boiling point and then steamed under pressure; this pressure forces some of the nutritional material from the bran layer into the inner rice grain. Converted (parboiled) rice then has greater nutritional value than does ordinary white rice.

Sodium/Caloric Content of Rice

One ounce of brown rice has 3 mg of sodium; one ounce of converted rice has 6 mg of sodium; and one ounce of white rice has less than 1 mg of sodium—so the trade-off in nutritive content is balanced by a lower sodium content. (These values are for rice cooked in water to which *no salt* has been added.)

One cup of cooked brown rice has 200 calories; one cup of cooked converted rice has 188 calories; one cup of cooked white rice has only 184 calories. Here again, loss of nutrients is balanced by fewer calories.

Rice as a Good Diet Food

Supermarkets offer a wide variety of rice products as well as the three varieties of the grain itself. There are rice breakfast cereals, rice flours, and even wines made from rice. One particularly interesting rice product is the rice cake, which is a valuable replacement for junk-food snacks. It comes in chewy four-inch wafers that are free of salt and cholesterol and contain only thirty-five calories per wafer. One excellent version is made of whole-grain brown rice with sesame seeds. Rice cakes have the advantage of being good for you at the same time that they satisfy your hunger.

Although Duke University's rice diet is effective, one of the most important reasons that its use is not more widespread can be traced to the development of various medications that reduce blood pressure, regardless of diet, or to drugs known as diuretic agents that enable the kidneys to lose salt, thereby producing an effect within the body similar to that produced by a reduction of salt in the diet. Perhaps the rice diet is too vigorous an approach and too difficult to maintain for most people, but fortunately the choice is not just between medication and the rice diet. Other options are available, as you will learn from this book.

9 ∼∼∼

Cholesterol as a Culprit

Aware that she was late for a business appointment, Debra was sprinting for a bus when she suddenly felt a sharp pain, as if someone had put arms around her chest and started to squeeze. As she staggered under this crushing sensation, she began having trouble breathing. She could not seem to draw in enough air. She collapsed on the ground and lay back, gasping. A passerby, noticing her distress, called the police, and moments later a medical team arrived. They gave Debra oxygen and intravenous fluid, and as soon as she was in the ambulance, they attached an electrocardiograph. It revealed that one area of her heart no longer produced a normal electrical pattern. This area, cut off from its blood supply; was dead. Debra had suffered a kind of heart attack that is known as a myocardial infarction.

The Different Types of Heart Attacks

Heart attacks can be as sudden and dramatic as the one described above—or silent and painless. Millions have suffered heart attacks and never been aware of them. Indications of previous heart attacks are often found during autopsies of persons who die from disorders other than cardiac problems but whose overall physical condition has not been greatly affected by weakening of their heart muscles.

High blood pressure is a leading culprit in causing heart disease, particularly the excruciating chest pains known as angina pectoris.

In addition to increasing the danger of heart attacks, one of this country's leading killers, hypertension is also a major risk factor in strokes and other serious ailments already discussed in Chapter 3. An important connection has been found between cholesterol, on the one hand, and life-threatening diseases and high blood pressure, on the other.

Cholesterol's Contribution

In appearance, cholesterol is a soapy, yellowish-white type of fat that is an essential body-building block. It is the envelope that surrounds our body cells. It is found in bile, in the insulation of the nerves, and as a component of androgen (the male sex hormone) and estrogen (the female sex hormone). The body can manufacture cholesterol with ease, but about 25 percent of the cholesterol in the body comes from what we eat.

Excess cholesterol is carried in the blood and deposited in the walls of the arteries. Ultimately this action produces a condition known as arteriosclerosis, in which the blood flow in the arteries is blocked, causing, among other things, a heart attack.

A diet high in saturated fat increases blood cholesterol by as much as 25 percent. Saturated fat is transformed in the liver into cholesterol. Therefore, to decrease the blood cholesterol level, you must decrease the level of saturated fat in your diet. Unsaturated fat does not change to cholesterol as does saturated fat, but actually produces a reduction in blood cholesterol.

How Much Is Too Much?

The average American consumes about 450 mg of cholesterol each day—not hard to do when you consider that one egg has 247 mg of cholesterol plus 1.7 mg of saturated fats that will be transformed into more cholesterol! This figure is far too high, especially for those men and women in their early forties who have cholesterol levels of 260 ml/dl as well as for about half the population whose levels are above the acceptable 200 ml/dl.

The importance of dietary control increases as cholesterol levels rise, or even if they are simply found to be high. The table on pages 104–105 shows the cholesterol content of many of the foods we eat. A change in diet to reduce the consumption of high-cholesterol foods, substituting safer foods such as fresh fruits, vegetables, grains, chicken, and fish while reducing the intake of saturated fats such as ice cream, is essential. Although a change in diet is urgent, important, and possibly life-saving, diet alone can control only a portion of the cholesterol level in the blood. In fact, it is possible that only a 15 percent reduction in cholesterol levels can be accomplished by limiting what you eat.

HDL to the Rescue

HDL is medical shorthand for the "high-density lipo-proteins" that help your body in its battle with choles-terol.

The cholesterol carried in the bloodstream takes different molecular forms, and those forms are impor-tant to the development of arteriosclerosis. Choles-terol is contained in minute circular packages of fat that are enclosed within a protein envelope. This com-bination is called a lipoprotein. Lipoproteins are clas-sified as *low-density lipoproteins* or *high-density lipoproteins*, depending on the amount of fat they con-tain.

The amount of fat or lipid carried within the protein envelope determines whether it will cause arterioscle-rosis or prevent it from occurring. Low-density lipo-proteins (LDL) are composed mainly of cholesterol and, therefore, their action in the body is bad. High-density lipoproteins (HDL) are mainly protein; their action in the body is good.

The LDL fat envelopes are the ones responsible for the deposition of cholesterol on the arterial walls. The HDL envelopes, on the other hand, draw the choles-terol/fat away from the walls of the arteries.

Although differences of opinion about HDL exist among experts, there seems to be agreement on the following points:

- HDL is low in sedentary males, in obese per-sons, and in patients with diabetes.
- HDL is high in women of childbearing age and in marathon runners.
- Exercise will increase the level of HDL.

Fat and Cholesterol in Selected Foods*

100-gm Edible Serving	Total Fat (gm)	Cholesterol (mg)
Beef approx. 6% fat, cooked	6.10	91.0
Beef approx. 30% fat, cooked	32.00	94.0
Lamb approx. 7% fat, cooked	7.00	100.0
Lamb approx. 30% fat, cooked	29.40	98.0
Veal approx. 6% fat, cooked	6.70	99.0
Veal approx. 25% fat, cooked	25.20	101.0
Chicken, turkey, Cornish hen, light meat with skin	3.40	78.0
Duck, goose (domestic) without skin	8.20	91.0
Beef, ground, fat unknown	32.00	94.0
Beef bologna	30.00	52.0
Pork, fresh, 30% fat, cooked	30.60	89.0
Frankfurter, all beef, cooked	30.00	51.0
Frankfurter, type unknown	27.20	62.0
Smoked pork, 25% fat, cooked	25.70	89.0
Bologna, salami, cold cuts, 25% fat	27.50	91.5
Bacon, regular, cooked	52.00	79.0
Cold cuts, variety unknown	27.50	91.5
Turkey frankfurters	23.76	98.5
Fish, 6% fat	4.00	66.0
Fish, 12% fat	13.40	84.0
Herring, canned, smoked, pickled	13.60	97.0
Salmon, pink, canned	5.90	35.0
Sardines, canned, drained	11.10	140.0
Tuna, canned, oil packed, drained	8.20	65.0
Tuna, canned, water packed	0.80	63.0
Clams, cooked	2.50	63.0
Crabmeat, cooked, canned	2.50	101.0
Crab, soft shell, steamed	2.50	100.0
Lobster, cooked	1.50	85.0
Oysters, cooked	2.20	45.0
Scallops, cooked	1.40	53.0
Shrimp, cooked	1.10	150.0
Caviar	15.00	300.0
Eggs, whole	11.50	504.0
Egg, yolk	30.60	1,480.0
Egg, white	—	—
Egg substitute, brand unknown	9.50	3.4
Creamer, imitation, liquid, frozen, saturated vegetable fat	11.00	0
Creamer—Poly Perx	10.00	0

Fat and Cholesterol in Selected Foods*

100-gm Edible Serving	Total Fat (gm)	Cholesterol (mg)
Cream, light, sweet or sour, 20% fat	20.60	66.0
Buttermilk, 1% fat	0.80	2.3
Milk, 1% fat	1.00	2.9
Milk, 2% fat	2.00	5.8
Milk, whole	3.50	13.5
Cheese—grated, dry, creamed	26.50	95.0
cottage, low salt	2.00	8.3
cottage, creamed	4.20	14.7
cream, Neufchatel, 20% fat	21.18	76.0
cheddar, American, blue, feta, Liederkranz, Camembert	32.20	102.4
Yogurt—part skim, plain	1.70	7.0
part skim, all flavors	0.85	4.6
whole milk, all flavors	3.40	13.2
Ice cream, medium rich, 16% fat	16.10	57.0
Sherbet	1.20	3.5
Ice milk	5.10	14.4
Oil—corn	100.00	0
cottonseed	100.00	0
safflower	100.00	0
sesame	100.00	0
soybean, partially hydrogenated	100.00	0
olive	100.00	0
peanut	100.00	0
coconut	100.00	0
palm	100.00	0
Shortening, household, vegetable	100.00	0
Margarine—% fat unknown—tub	81.00	0
% fat unknown—stick	17.70	0
Mayonnaise, commercial or homemade	79.90	70.0
Peanut butter	50.60	0
Almonds	54.20	0
Cashews	45.70	0
Peanuts	48.70	0
Walnuts	64.00	0
Olives, black	13.80	0
Lard, rendered	100.00	95.0
Butter, sweet or salted	81.00	227.3

*Adapted from data provided by The Nutrition Coding Center, University of Minnesota. Supported by Contract No. 1-HV-6-2941-L of the National Heart, Lung, and Blood Institute.

- Diet can help reduce LDL but does not affect HDL.
- Monounsaturated fats such as olive and peanut oil may help to lower LDL but do not affect HDL.

You can apply these findings to your own life by (1) avoiding excess weight; (2) exercising regularly; and (3) avoiding saturated fats. The goal is to raise HDL levels and lower LDL levels.

Anticholesterol Medications

A new drug, Questran or cholestyramine resin, was recently introduced to reduce blood cholesterol levels. Its use should be accompanied by a low-cholesterol diet. There are side effects to this medication, so it is important to rule out other causes for high blood cholesterol levels, such as diabetes or thyroid problems, before administering cholestyramine. I also advise trying a low-cholesterol diet along with a weight-reduction plan before resorting to this drug. Constipation is the most common side effect of Questran. Others include nausea, vomiting, GI (gastrointestinal) upset, GI bleeding, and diarrhea.

What Animal Experiments Have Shown

Laboratory experiments have shown a direct correlation between a diet high in cholesterol and elevations in blood pressure. Very importantly, other experiments showed that, in turn, hypertension itself increased the cholesterol level in the blood. We do not know exactly how hypertension increases cholesterol. Probably the cholesterol enters the walls of the arteries, making them more rigid and resistant to expansion. This would increase blood flow resistance, and pressure would rise.

In other words, cholesterol and hypertension each contribute to rising rates of the other. And since each is such a deadly force in the lives it touches, you should keep the connection in mind, especially when it comes to your easily controllable life-style.

10 ≈

The Role of Potassium and Calcium in High Blood Pressure

The Positive Part Potassium May Play

In 1982, Dr. George R. Meenely and Dr. Harold R. Batterbee of the Louisiana State University Medical Center at Shreveport reported on a link between potassium and high blood pressure. In experiments with rats, Meenely and Batterbee found that potassium helped *protect against* an increase in blood pressure caused by excess sodium (salt). Other studies suggest that potassium may offer similar protection in human beings.

Potassium is a chemical component that has a great many properties similar to sodium, and the two are interrelated in the complex mechanisms by which the body functions. Potassium is the chemical within the body cells, whereas sodium is the major chemical in the fluid between and around the cells.

Nature has put potassium in so many foods that it is almost impossible to have a diet deficient in it. Futhermore, it is so well controlled by the body—excreted with such ease—that excessive intake has no ill effects on the healthy individual.

In certain disease states, however, too much potassium can cause trouble. For example, in kidney disease, where potassium is not adequately excreted, excess potassium can cause serious complications. In such people, dietary control of potassium is necessary. Because of this, some experts feel that the potassium content of common foods should be listed along with the sodium content.

When Is Extra Potassium Needed?

Some people require extra potassium because their bodies lose too much of this chemical. This is true for those people taking antihypertensive diuretics that produce excessive urination to remove sodium from the body. In these cases, potassium also is removed, and it must be replaced to keep the body's chemicals in balance. The most widely used foods for this purpose are bananas and bouillon cubes. (Low-sodium bouillon cubes are available.) Some people may also require potassium tablets to make up for the deficiency.

There are a few other disease processes that cause a deficiency of potassium. The most common direct cause of potassium loss is from the intestinal tract as a result of diarrhea or vomiting. However, the normal person who is on a regular diet and not taking antihypertensive medications should not have a deficiency of potassium because the average diet is so rich in this

Foods High in Potassium
for Potassium Supplementation

Food	Average Serving	Potassium (mg)
Apricots		
canned	½ cup	239
dried, uncooked	30 halves	979
fresh	3 small	281
Asparagus		
frozen	app. ½ cup	239
Avocados	½	604
Banana	1 medium	370
Beans, lima		
fresh, cooked	½ cup	422
frozen, cooked	½ cup	394
Beef	3⅓ oz.	370
Beet greens, cooked	½ cup	332
Beets, fresh, boiled	½ cup	208
Broccoli	⅔ cup	267
Brussel sprouts	¾ cup	273
Buttermilk	8 oz (240 gm)	336
Cabbage, raw, average	1 cup or ⅓ small	265
Candy, chocolate		
milk, plain	3 oz	384
with almonds	3 oz	442
with peanuts	3 oz	487
semisweet	3 oz	325
Carrots, fresh, cooked	⅔ cup	222
Caramels	3 oz	192
Cauliflower	1 cup	206
Chard, Swiss, boiled	½ cup	321
Chicken		
dark	3⅓ oz	321
white	3⅓ oz	411
Chocolate beverage drink		
commercial, with skim milk	8 oz	341
hot chocolate, homemade	8 oz	355
Cider	8 oz	242
Collards, cooked	½ cup	234
Cookies		
gingersnaps (50 gm)	12 small	231
macaroons	5 large	463
oatmeal w/raisins	4 large	370

Foods High In Potassium
for Potassium Supplimentation (continued)

Food	Average Serving	Potassium (mg)
Cowpeas, cooked	½ cup	379
Crackers, graham-plain	5 squares	384
Dates, dried	12	684
Duck	3⅓ oz	285
Figs, dried	12	640
Fish, average	3⅓ oz	390
Goose	3⅓ oz	605
Grapefruit juice	8 oz	389
Grapefruit sections	1 cup	346
Grape juice	8 oz	278
Lamb	3⅓ oz	290
Malted milk	8 oz	480
Mango	2 small	378
Milk		
evaporated	8 oz	727
skim	8 oz	348
whole	8 oz	346
Mushrooms, raw	½ cup	414
Mustard greens, boiled	½ cup	220
Nectarines	2 medium	294
Nuts—unsalted		
Brazil	20	715
cashew	20	464
filberts	60	704
peanuts, roasted with skin	50	701
walnuts, halved	1 cup	460
Orange	1 medium	200
Orange juice, all kinds	8 oz	480
Orange and grapefruit juice	8 oz	442
Papaya	¼ medium	234
Parsnips	½ cup or ½ medium	379
Peaches, fresh	1 medium	202
Peanut butter	2 tablespoons	250
Peas, fresh	½ cup	196
Pies		
coconut custard	⅙ of 9″ pie	244
custard	⅙ of 9″ pie	206
peach	⅙ of 9″ pie	224
pumpkin	⅙ of 9″ pie	240
rhubarb	⅙ of 9″ pie	239

Foods High In Potassium for Potassium Supplementation (continued)		
Food	Average Serving	Potassium (mg)
Pineapple juice	8 oz	358
Plums, damson—raw	2 medium	299
Pomegranate	2 small	259
Pork	3⅓ oz	390
Potato, white		
baked in skin	1 medium	503
boiled without skin	1 medium	285
french fried	20 pcs	853
mashed with milk	½ cup	261
Prunes, uncooked	20	940
Prune juice	8 oz	564
Raisins	¾ cup	763
Rutabagas, cooked	¾ cup	250
Salsify, cooked	½ cup	266

element. The table on pages 110–112 shows many of the foods that are high in this mineral.

The National Academy of Science's Food and Nutrition Board, which establishes recommended daily allowances for essential nutrients, suggests that adults consume between 1,875 and 5,625 mg of potassium each day.

Calcium's Contribution

Calcium is basic to our bone structure. It is also essential to our teeth, giving them the solid consistency needed to chew food. It plays an important role in blood clotting, too; without calcium, bleeding cannot be stopped. Finally, calcium is essential to our nervous system and to the normal functioning of body cells. The body is believed to require calcium in amounts ranging from 400 mg to 1,300 mg a day.

The chief sources of calcium are milk and milk products, dark green vegetables, and shellfish (see table below for some comparative figures). Calcium cannot get into the body if there is a deficiency of vitamin D or if there is inadequate exposure to the sun.

Calcium Content of Various Foods		
	Amount	*mg*
Dairy		
Whole milk	1 cup	288
Skim milk	1 cup	296
Swiss cheese	1 oz	262
Ice cream	½ cup	97
Vegetables (raw)*		
Broccoli	3½ oz	103
Collard greens	3½ oz	203
Kale	3½ oz	179
Parsley	3½ oz	203
Tomato	3½ oz	13
Turnip greens	3½ oz	246
Fruit*		
Grapefruit	3½ oz	16
Cantaloupe	3½ oz	14

*Cooking diminishes the calcium content of vegetables. For example, 3½ oz of cooked kale contain 134 mg of calcium as opposed to 179 mg raw; cooked turnip greens have 184 mg of calcium but 246 mg raw.
†Fruit generally has little or no calcium—grapefruit and cantaloupe are the two best bets.

Calcium Loss as a Factor in Hypertension

Too little calcium in the diet may be a little-recognized factor contributing to high blood pressure, according to a study conducted at Oregon Health Sciences University in Portland (*Science* 217:267–69, 1982). These researchers found that the amounts of milk and non-dairy products containing calcium were present in equal quantities in hypertensives and in those who were not hypertensive, but that the hypertensives consumed fewer dairy products other than milk than did people with normal blood pressure.

David A. McCarron, M.D., an associate professor of medicine and director of the hypertension program at Oregon Health Sciences University, thinks that calcium is *the* answer to the cause of hypertension. He says the passage of calcium into and out of cells brings about the degree of tightness that determines the blood pressure within our arteries. When there is a shortage of calcium, relaxation of the artery walls is insufficient, and the result is hypertension. The findings are not altogether convincing, but they have caught on in the medical community.

Since about 60 to 70 percent of our calcium comes from dairy products—milk, cheese, ice cream—Dr. McCarron feels that eliminating dairy products from the diet results in an insufficient supply of calcium in the body. When he surveyed forty-seven hypertensives and forty-four people with normal blood pressure to discover what they were eating, he found that all the hypertensives were getting less than the minimum daily requirement of calcium.

In my opinion, these findings, while interesting, are not convincing. This type of dietary evaluation cannot be proved with enough accuracy to be called fact. In addition, the number of people in the McCarron survey was far too small to be applicable to hypertensives everywhere.

The human body contains more calcium than any other of the essential minerals—an essential mineral being one that the body requires in amounts greater than 100 mg a day. Everyone has about 1,500 g of calcium, most of it in the bones. It does not make sense that a decrease in the recommended daily allowance of 800 mg would be a basic cause of high blood pressure, since the body has such a large reserve to balance the reduction.

Other Effects of Calcium Loss

In older people a loss of calcium causes their bones to weaken and soften, a condition called osteoporosis; this is particularly prevalent in women past the menopause.

Long periods of bed rest will also cause loss of calcium from the bones. People who have broken a hip and cannot move around may find it difficult to regain easy use of their limbs as a result of calcium loss produced by lack of body motion.

Effects of Too Much Calcium

Intakes of larger amounts of calcium (2,500 mg per day) may not cause problems for healthy individuals, but for people with kidney disease, a large intake of calcium can produce serious complications.

Some people develop kidney stones when they have an excessive amount of calcium. We do not know why this occurs in some people and not in others, but excessive absorption of calcium into the body is a basic cause.

Kidney stones are a fairly common problem. They

often start with severe pain, called renal colic, although at times they can be painless. Since stones can destroy the kidney, once they are discovered they require hospital care and, frequently, surgery.

The Final Word Is Yet to Come

Until recently there was no satisfactory medication to help prevent the formation of kidney stones. Recently the Food and Drug Administration approved a medication that draws calcium from the intestinal tract so that the body cannot absorb the calcium.

Because this medication is new, we are not yet familiar with all its potential side effects. Will it cause osteoporosis? Will patients taking it develop hypertension? For those researchers who believe that calcium reduction underlies hypertension, it is possible that experience with the use of this drug may lead to further confirmation of their theories.

III

YOUR STYLE OF LIVING

~~~~~~

You won't have to depend on medicines so much if you learn some new habits and discard a couple of old ones. Such as? Learn to exercise and use relaxation techniques; get rid of cigarettes and alcohol.

11

Smoke Gets in Your Blood

There is every reason to believe that smoking, which is really nothing less than taking a toxic substance into the body, has an ill effect on both blood pressure and the heart.

Smoking can produce a significant rise in the pulse rate as well as in the systolic and diastolic blood pressure, according to Dr. Philip E. Cryer of the Washington University School of Medicine in St. Louis. In an article in the September 1976 *New England Journal of Medicine*, he reported that within 2.5 minutes after a person started to smoke there was a rise in the pulse rate; systolic pressure increased by a total of about 12 points, as did diastolic pressure. In his study, a similar rise in pressure and pulse rate did not occur in a control group given placebo cigarettes.

These findings clearly indicate that anyone with high blood pressure—and anyone who wishes to avoid having it—should stop smoking.

At present about 30 percent of Americans smoke. Among this extremely large number are many people who would like to stop but feel they can't. Perhaps you are one of them.

What are the chances that if you want to stop you will finally be successful? According to government studies, about 40 percent of the smokers who want to stop will do so if they are sufficiently motivated and if they receive professional help. One of the most effective initial aids in getting people to stop smoking is their physician's suggestion that they should do so, probably because this advice taps right into their own realization that smoking is impairing their health.

Withdrawal from Nicotine Isn't Easy

Today smoking is recognized to result from an addiction to nicotine. Nicotine increases the brain's electrical activity via an arousal-type reaction; the brain's response to nicotine results in a sense of intensified satisfaction. In order to quit, therefore, you must have sufficient self-control and willpower to overcome the withdrawal effects of the drug, for these withdrawal effects take the form of a need for repeated exposure —the famous "just one more cigarette." For the truly addicted, willpower alone is not enough, and additional supportive measures are necessary.

Although many smokers can control the degree of nicotine intake by shortening the extent and frequency of the "drag," or inhalation of smoke, quitting "cold turkey" is believed to be easier than a gradual reduction or "slow stop" because the withdrawal symptoms subside more rapidly when the cutoff is sudden.

The ability to cope with withdrawal symptoms varies, depending on the individual. Some people can tolerate the discomfort, while others cannot. Obviously, those who cannot deal with the withdrawal symptoms will quickly return to smoking unless they seek some help. However, the degree of tolerance can often be measured against the motivation to quit—which can be said about any addiction, including alcoholism. In the end, motivation is the most basic factor to success.

Nicotine Dependence

I do not believe that all smokers are as nicotine-dependent as various studies would suggest. Just as there are social drinkers in contradistinction to true alcoholics, so there are some smokers for whom the compulsion to smoke is less compelling than it is for others. My own response to smoking was never as intense as a true nicotine dependence would have been. Because my smoking was nonaddictive and rather uncomplex, I found quitting relatively simple, unlike the heavy smoker who, being nicotine-dependent, finds it extremely difficult.

For me, smoking was an activity that occupied my hands while I was thinking. I recognized that often I smoked while I was working on a book or an article. When I stopped to decide what I was going to write next, I would take my hands off the typewriter keyboard and light a cigarette as a diversion while I thought. The lighting-up process provided just the right amount of time to organize my thoughts. However, once I made that connection and understood what I was doing, I was able to retrain myself to sit at the typewriter and think with my hands resting on the typing table instead of lighting up a cigarette. Today I don't miss smoking at all.

How to Stop

Here's the approach I recommend to my patients who want to kick the cigarette habit:

As a first step, try to go it alone. Although this method for giving up smoking *seems* the least complicated and the easiest, it may actually prove to be the most difficult. However, start out with the determination that you are going to have sufficient willpower to make a "dead stop." Throw out the cigarette habit literally by putting your remaining cigarettes in the garbage pail.

This was the method I used about ten years ago. I made up my mind one day that I would stop, and I did, although it was not always easy. Fortunately, on those occasions when I wanted to start smoking again (and at first they were frequent), I had the necessary self-control not to give way.

I remember one extremely difficult situation when I almost backslid—it was the moment when I had to give a patient the results of some tests, and the news was bad. Telling people that they are seriously ill is no simple matter. In this particular instance I sat at the bedside of a very young man and started to tell him about the severity of his illness and the fact that he would need a very radical kind of surgery. As I presented the unpleasant facts to him, he reached into the bedside table drawer and took out a fresh pack of cigarettes, a brand I was accustomed to smoking. He opened it and offered me a cigarette. I guess the need to supply myself with the emotional "lift" of nicotine was great, for I started to reach for the cigarette and then got control of myself. I said "No, thanks" and advised him that he should give up smoking, too. That incident has stayed with me, for from then on I knew I would never return to smoking.

If you wish to go it alone, the American Cancer Society provides an excellent self-help kit as part of its Stop Smoking Program. It contains six sections—Why Quit. How Quit. When Quit. Who Quit. We Quit. Stay Quit—and presents the many aspects of giving up smoking in a very interesting manner.

When You Need Help

It isn't always possible—or even advisable—to go the do-it-yourself route. Special techniques and support measures may be necessary for some people. If this is your situation, seek professional help, which is readily available in any large city. Many organizations sponsor groups that will help you stop smoking permanently. The American Cancer Society has numerous groups, all based on behavior modification followed by peer-support methods. The groups meet about twice a week for six to ten sessions. There are also a number of ex-smokers' clubs to help keep you smoking-free.

The various state lung associations also offer courses that use peer support and behavior modification. Other groups that offer help are the Seventh-Day Adventists, and Smokenders (50 Washington Street, Norwalk, Conn.).

Hypnosis seminars and acupuncture are other methods that have been used to combat smoking. Another rather simple aid is nicotine gum, a chewing gum that contains 2 mg of nicotine and can be used as a "tapering off" measure to replace the nicotine obtained from cigarettes. Some initial studies indicate that a good percentage of the people who use this gum are helped considerably. It is particularly valuable for people who quit smoking cold turkey.

Helping the Hard-Core Smoker

In the *New York State Journal of Medicine* (1982), Drs. D. R. Powell and C. B. Arnold described a five-day stop-smoking multiple-treatment program used to help twenty-two men with an increased risk of coronary artery disease. They were considered hard-core smokers because they had failed to quit after five years of continuous effort.

The program taught them new skills to combat smoking. The techniques seem to work, because one year after treatment 50 percent were still smoke-free. The degree of success was not gauged by the testimony of the smoker who says he has quit, but rather by blood studies. The blood of people who smoke contains a chemical—serum thiocyanate—that varies in proportion to the number of cigarettes smoked. Within fourteen days of cessation of smoking, half the total amount of serum thiocyanate is gone from the blood. In the people in this study, the levels soon fell from a high to a normal range.

The study concluded that various techniques emphasizing behavior modification effectively helped this group of high-risk patients stop smoking permanently, which they had previously been unable to do on their own.

The methods of therapy used in this study included the following behavior-modification and self-control techniques:

1. *Stimulus control: the altering of smoking antecedents*.

This means that you remove those factors that cause you to want to take a cigarette. For example, if you always take a cigarette when you sit down to watch TV, replace the cigarette with a cup of tea, or hold a newspaper instead of taking a cigarette.

2. *Relaxation training: the use of deep-breathing exercises and pleasant mental imagery to reduce the stress associated with cravings.*
   Instead of taking a cigarette, stand up and do some deep-breathing exercises. Think about something pleasant to allay your anxiety.

3. *Thought-stopping: a procedure that extinguishes repetitive thoughts about smoking.*
   Don't say to yourself, "I need a smoke." Replace that idea with something like, "If others can do without the weed, so can I."

4. *Eating management: avoidance of foods and eating situations that trigger the desire to smoke.*
   Don't sit down on your coffee break and pick up a cigarette. Change the entire pattern by eating an apple instead. Understand that you are deliberately doing this *instead* of smoking a cigarette.

5. *Incompatible behavior: the use of oral and manual substitutes such as sugar-free candies and binder clips when the urge to smoke occurs.*
   If you are eating candy or chewing on something, you cannot very easily smoke. A binder clip is a small clip that goes on your lips when you feel the urge to smoke.

6. *Behavior rehearsal: imagination of desired nonsmoking behavior.*

7. *Cognitive coping: procedures for thinking positively about the quitting experience.*
   See each day without cigarettes as a positive achievement in willpower and health.

These methods work, but more important than the individual success of these particular techniques is the knowledge that treatment in general can be effective. There is hope for even the most resistant smoker.

Cigarettes and Your Weight

Many people are concerned that they will gain weight if they stop smoking—a valid worry, since excess weight is a health concern, too. However, you do not have to gain if you understand the problem. After they stop smoking, the people who gain weight do so because they eat to overcome nicotine withdrawal symptoms. They use food as a substitute for cigarettes. If you have self-awareness, you can avoid this problem by meeting these cravings with various low-calorie snacks or low-calorie, low-salt sodas or by substituting activities for eating.

Smoke of a Different Color

I had an interesting experience with a young woman recently. She had been admitted to the hospital because of kidney stones. Although she was only twenty-two and quite slim, a medical exam showed her to have very high blood pressure. We could find no cause for such a high reading despite numerous tests, and we eventually concluded that she had what is commonly called "essential hypertension"—high blood pressure due to no known cause.

But in the course of my treatment, she happened to mention that she usually smoked at least a joint of marijuana, sometimes even two or three, each day. Now, of course, in the hospital she had no access to this sort of drug, and I began to notice that her blood pressure gradually started to drop.

I saw her for several months of continued treatment after her release from the hospital, and her blood pressure remained normal. She told me she had given up pot.

There is yet no fully corroborated scientific evidence regarding the correlation between use of marijuana and high blood pressure, but this case struck me as pertinent and important. If *you* indulge, get your pressure checked by your doctor.

12 ≈≈≈

How Alcohol Accelerates Hypertension

The relationship between hypertension and excessive alcohol consumption has been recognized for the past seventy years. During this time, repeated scientific studies have confirmed that alcoholism is a cause of hypertension. This connection is independent of any other factors, such as socioeconomic status, age, race, weight, serum cholesterol levels, or tobacco use. If you drink excessively, your blood pressure will go up.

Which Comes First?

Just how this works is not yet established. It is possible that it is a reverse relationship—that hypertension occurs first and that excessive drinking follows as a result of a need for relief from internal pressure; for example, certain driven and success-oriented people might develop hypertension and then turn to drinking to relax.

Do Genes Play a Part?

It has also been suggested that there might be a genetic predisposition to both hypertension and alcoholism. If so, how could one structure a study to determine the validity of this theory? One way might be to study a group of twins who had the same genetic background but were raised separately. You would then need to have one twin who drinks and one who does not. On the surface, these sound like impossible conditions. However, just such a study was conducted in 1974 in Sweden, where seventy pairs of male twins were studied. Each twin had been raised separately from the other. Blood-pressure levels and alcohol-consumption levels were compared for each set of twins, and it was found that the blood-pressure reading was invariably higher in the twin who drank.

The results of this study would indicate that the hypertension that accompanies alcoholism is an alcohol-induced rather than a genetically inherited trait. However, despite the fact that finding seventy pairs of twins who fit the requirements seems an achievement in itself, for scientific purposes the number of people in this study is too small to be definitive, so the genetic factor cannot be ruled out. (When I first reviewed this study, I thought it was remarkable that the investigator had been able to find 70 pairs of twins who had been raised separately. Then it occurred to me that one of my own adopted children is one of a pair of twins who were separated at birth and raised apart.)

Effects in Long-Term Drinkers

The effect of drinking on hypertension has been proved over and over again, even if the exact reason for the connection has not yet been established. Various studies in England and Wales demonstrated that long-term drinking invariably leads to hypertension and its various severe complications, such as strokes and heart attacks. Another European study showed that the death rate from strokes was three times greater in heavy drinkers than in infrequent drinkers. In this study, high blood pressure was the cause of strokes among heavy drinkers, underlining the link between alcohol and high blood pressure.

In the United States a study of twenty-five hundred men and an equal number of women revealed that elevated blood pressure was directly related to the amount of alcohol consumed. Other studies, involving equally large numbers of people, confirmed that alcohol consumption was an important factor in elevated blood pressure. In these studies, the blood-pressure levels of people who drank sixty ounces of hard liquor per month were twice those of persons who drank less than thirty ounces of hard liquor a month.

Other Health Concerns

Certainly there is more than ample proof that alcohol causes hypertension, a finding of extreme importance in view of the fact that hypertension can lead to strokes, heart attacks, and various other serious disorders. The problem of alcoholism has a bearing on the health and well-being of millions of Americans as well as great economic impact on ballooning health-care costs.

Ironically, a December 1983 report titled "The Fifth Special Report to the U.S. Congress on Alcohol and Health," made to the Congress of the United States by the Department of Health and Human Services, does not mention the connection between alcohol and hypertension. The report includes a long section titled "The Medical Consequences of Alcohol," yet nowhere does it refer to alcohol's role in causing hypertension —an inexplicable oversight in view of the fact that its harmful effect is common knowledge in the medical community.

Clinical Experience

Even if all the scientific studies did not confirm that alcohol causes hypertension, you need only ask practicing physicians what their experience has been. Most will acknowledge that when patients describe a pattern of heavy drinking, subsequent examination will reveal that they have high blood pressure.

Intellectual ability and special talent are no protections here. One patient of mine, a gifted writer and foreign correspondent whose reports on various overseas assignments were brilliant, suffered from disastrously high blood pressure and was repeatedly warned about drinking. Nonetheless, as soon as he got home, he would go on periodic binges. I was often called to his home when he was in a state of delirium, seeing the classic "pink elephants." When he was sober, no amount of discussion could convince him of the self-destruction involved in his drinking. He continued to drink despite rising blood pressure levels until he was too sick to travel or work.

Physiological Effects of Alcohol

The body of the heavy drinker takes a severe beating. The organ most frequently damaged is the *liver*, because the liver is responsible for getting alcohol out of the system. When excessive amounts of alcohol become concentrated in the liver, they cause great damage. The liver must try to burn off alcohol instead of fat; as a result, the liver becomes infiltrated with fat, which leads first to hepatitis or inflammation of the liver, and finally to cirrhosis or total destruction of the liver.

Because a properly functioning liver destroys many toxins in the body, when the liver itself is being destroyed, many other systems also become unbalanced. A healthy liver destroys unneeded hormones; when it is not functioning properly, hormonal imbalances occur. Concomitant nutritional imbalances occur as well.

Alcohol also causes the personality to fall into disarray and can destroy the functioning of the *nervous system*. How does this happen? Normally the brain cells, or neurons, communicate with one another via electrical impulses or by the passage of various chemical molecules that act as messengers. These impulses and molecules pass from cell to cell, moving within the liquid medium of each cell. When alcohol is absorbed into this liquid, it produces physical changes. The viscosity or thickness of the fluid is altered so that the passage of electrical impulses and molecules is delayed, slowed, or even prevented. This obstruction accounts for the depression of brain activity; when drinking persists, the changes that occur in the liquid medium are more permanent. It is possible that long-term damage to the nervous system is a reason for the development of hypertension, as we shall shortly see.

How Does Alcohol Affect Blood Pressure?

We understand the mechanism by which the liver is destroyed. We are aware of the effects of alcohol on the brain and the nervous system. But what is the mechanism that causes the blood pressure to rise? Although the exact cause is not known, our knowledge of the damage alcohol does to the nervous system provides some clues.

Injury to the nervous system can result in an imbalance in the hormones that control blood pressure. When the nerves that regulate the production of hormones are damaged by alcohol and fail to function properly, the kidneys and adrenal glands, which produce the hormones that raise the level of the blood pressure, are given no signal to stop, and therefore they overproduce. This overproduction is a response to nerve damage rather than to an actual lack of hormones—an example of a feedback system that is out of kilter. This hormonal overproduction may cause hypertension by elevating the blood pressure.

In beer drinkers, hypertension is often simply the result of the large amount of sodium in beer, since, as we know, too much sodium produces an increase in blood pressure. The amount of sodium contained in six beers is sufficient to raise the blood pressure in persons who are sodium-sensitive.

How Much Is Too Much?

Just how much alcohol does a person have to consume daily to be called a heavy drinker? A heavy drinker consumes 13 g of alcohol daily. You ingest this much alcohol if you consume daily:

Amount	Alcohol
5 or more 12-oz (360-ml) cans of beer	3.6% each
or	
5 or more drinks of 1.25 oz (375 ml), 80-proof whiskey	40.0% each
or	
5 or more 4-ounce (112-ml) glasses of wine	9.9% each

Although as yet there is not much experimental data to support it, the most reasonable explanation for the hypertension associated with drinking would seem to be attributable to the direct action of alcohol on the walls of the arteries. When alcohol is present in the bloodstream it actually bathes the walls of the blood vessels, increasing their tension and thereby causing high blood pressure.

There are other, more complex scientific explanations that tend to support this concept. According to one of them, alcohol blocks the normal passageway of chemicals into and out of the artery walls, resulting in the tightening of the walls. This tension produces a rise in blood pressure within the arteries.

There is little doubt that alcohol causes irritative phenomena that contribute to the rise in blood pressure. How else can one explain the fact that when a person stops drinking, the blood-pressure level decreases?

A Drinker's Questionnaire

How can you tell if you are an alcoholic? Finding a simple answer might seem difficult, but recent research conducted among large numbers of patients by Dr. John A. Ewing of the University of North Carolina at Chapel Hill has provided an excellent yardstick. He suggests that you answer the following four questions:

1. Have you ever felt you ought to cut down on your drinking?
2. Have people annoyed you by criticizing your drinking?
3. Have you ever felt bad or guilty about your drinking?
4. Have you ever had a drink first thing in the morning—an eye-opener to steady your nerves?

If you answer yes to two of these questions, then you are in the company of all the acknowledged alcoholics and 97 percent of the heavy drinkers in his study. Only 4 percent of the nonalcoholics in Ewing's study said that at some time in their lives they had thought they should decrease their drinking.

If you answered yes to three questions (which none of the nonalcoholics in the study did), you are in the same league as 95 percent of the alcoholics and 86 percent of the heavy drinkers. All the alcoholics in

Ewing's study thought they should cut down on their drinking.

An editorial in the October 12, 1984, issue of the *Journal of the American Medical Association*, an issue devoted to the problem of alcohol, encouraged physicians to check all drinkers for hypertension and to educate all hypertensives not to drink. The problem was well delineated in the editorial:

> Ethyl alcohol [alcohol] kills every day in Chicago, Los Angeles, New York, Paris and virtually every other city in the Western World. Considering all of its lethal effects, it follows right after heart disease, cancer and stroke as a cause of death.

It is important for anyone who drinks to get his or her blood pressure checked periodically, and it is extremely important for anyone with high blood pressure to stop drinking. The relationship is clearly established, and stopping has immediate benefits; studies have demonstrated that once you stop drinking, your high blood pressure as a result of drinking will invariably come down.

13 ~~

Stress and the Type A Personality

Stress and how you react to it can also determine whether you will have high blood pressure. Dealing with stress is often learned behavior that can be unlearned.

Mark's Case

Mark was one of the youngest students in the university's history. His reputation was unsurpassed, and to maintain it, he studied late into the night and devoted his hours after classes and his weekends to doing research. In his four years at school, he never had time to attend a dance or go to a football game. He often remarked that he could not understand why anyone would want to take a vacation when there was so much work to be done and so little time to do it.

Mark chose medical school after college, seeing it as

137

an opportunity to enhance his knowledge. In medical school he continued to devote all his waking hours to study, although, being a perfectionist, he thought that he was ill equipped to deal with many of life's problems and not sufficiently skilled to care for the sick. Confronted with this feeling of inferiority and the mistaken idea that he could not handle an internship, he chose to go to work for a large pharmaceutical company. He started as a drug monitor, a job that involved setting up the research for the development of new medications. His days often started at six in the morning and continued until late at night. His single-minded efforts resulted in the rapid approval of many of the company's new drugs.

About two months after a major promotion, he experienced some chest pains at the office. He refused to acknowledge them and, instead, continued to drive himself even harder, until the day he was stricken with a fatal heart attack—a tragic but not surprising ending to his high-pressured life.

Mark's story demonstrates some aspects of what is termed the type A personality, a designation coined by Meyer Friedman, M.D., in 1959 and presented in an article published in the *Journal of the American Medical Association*.

What Is the Type A Personality?

The type A personality is highly motivated, pressure-prone, constantly striving toward greater and greater accomplishments. He or she is aggressive, competitive, and very compulsive. This person is internally stressed, neither fun-loving nor interested in any of the pleasanter aspects of life. The type A personality is totally work-oriented.

At the other end of the behavior spectrum is the type B personality, an easygoing, low-keyed, laid-back individual, contemplative, relaxed, and often nonaggressive to the point of passivity. Unlike the type A personality, the type B personality is not internally stressed.

Type A and Hypertension

How do these two types react in a given situation? Let's take the case of two men, one type A, the other type B, who are almost hit by a car while crossing the street. Invariably, the type A personality will respond to this stress by showing a greater rise in blood pressure than does type B.

Does stress itself hold the key to hypertension? How important a role does the physiological reaction to stress play in the production of hypertension?

There are, of course, problems with an oversimplified concept of the type A and type B personalities. Most people are not pure A or pure B but rather a blend of both, with a greater propensity toward one or the other. While not all specialists agree on these types, there is certainly sufficient evidence to suggest that the theory has scientific merit.

How Can You Determine If You Are Type A or Type B?

1. Are you a hard-driving worker? Do you try to do more work than anyone else? Are you always striving to be recognized and rewarded for your accomplishments?

2. Do you feel that you *must* achieve? Do you pressure yourself to win awards?

3. Is time always against you? Do you feel there is never enough time to do all the things you want to do, that if only you could move faster you could do more?

4. Does it seem that everyone is after you to produce more work? Do you feel that no matter what you do, your boss always wants more done?

5. Do you feel that you must get ahead of everyone else? Are you competitive with everyone?

6. Do you find waiting in line for something so infuriating that you would rather do without it than endure the feelings of frustration?

7. Do you consider yourself a two-fisted, aggressive type?

If your answers are positive and you see yourself as a pressure-prone type A, it is time to consider the causes and try to alleviate them.

Inborn Traits

Anyone who has raised a number of children will tell you that some are born with a striving, driving personality that needs no outside motivation, while others are passive and easy-going and may not care to study or work. Although it is possible to change or mold several of these personality traits somewhat, most seem to remain essentially unchanged no matter how much one tries. Some people appear to be born with what might be called an internal stress factor, as differentiated from the naturally occurring external stress of daily life. The individual response to pressure is determined by the relationship between the degree of stress that is present externally and the internal stress that exists within the personality.

Defining Stress

The basic question, then, is: Can externally produced stress in itself cause hypertension? If one wishes to develop a method for treating or preventing hypertension without the use of medication, the answer to this question is extremely important, yet it is so complex that no single definitive statement can be made.

To understand this, let us consider what stress means. You will see that it is basically indefinable, or rather definable only for a single individual in a specific situation.

If I were to ask a group of people what they consider stressful situations, they probably would give a number of different answers:

- "When I can't pay my rent because I spent too much money during the month."
- "When I get caught in traffic and the car starts to overheat."
- "When I have to stand in line at the checkout counter after work."
- "When I get yelled at for not doing a better job with the dishes."
- "When my boss gives me a lot of typing at four-thirty and I have a five-o'clock date."
- "When I have to travel by plane."

141

The list is endless, for there are as many stressful situations as there are human beings, and the responses can be just as varied as the causes, since what may be stressful to one person is not to another.

Stress Is Universal

Although stress is a universally recognized phenomenon, it is difficult to define from a scientific point of view. Stress might best be described as an emotional tension superimposed on our psyche by conditions with which we believe we may be unable to cope. The result is anxiety. The basic cause is a high level of internal emotional pressure. When we talk about stress-induced hypertension, we are talking about something that is actually indefinable and unmeasurable.

Yet many experts continue to claim that stress causes hypertension. For example, an ad in *The New York Times* for Pfizer, Inc., a pharmaceuticals corporation, stated:

"What can be done about high blood pressure? Fortunately, plenty. First have regular checkups. Only your doctor can diagnose hypertension, but you can help head it off. Moderation is the key. Reduction in weight, cholesterol, salt intake, *stress* [italics added], anxiety, and smoking is the method" (Aug. 25, 1982).

Note that reduction of stress appears as one factor that can help control high blood pressure, a clear statement that stress can play a role in producing increased blood pressure.

Reaction to Stress Depends on the Person

The response to stress is highly individualized, as the following case histories demonstrate.

When Diana, a thirty-four-year-old stockbroker, came in for a routine medical exam, she had high blood pressure, although she said she felt fine and had had no symptoms.

I conducted an intensive medical investigation to try to determine why so young a woman should have such high blood pressure. When I couldn't find any medical cause, I made an extensive evaluation of her background and daily routine. Diana had been brought up in a very religious home and could best be described as conventional and rather hard on herself. She was slim and attractive and appeared to be in good overall health. She told me she never drank, although her Wall Street job involved some socializing and was very high-pressured. Every day she had to make far-reaching decisions that involved large sums of money. Any error in judgment could result in substantial losses, a failure that would be noted immediately.

In the absence of any other problems, it seemed to me that her stressful job clearly was the cause of the high blood pressure.

Yet I questioned this explanation a month later, when Diana referred her co-worker William to me. This man had blood pressure that was well below what is considered normal, yet he had exactly the same job as Diana. Their work was literally identical; they shared equally in making decisions and in the consequences of those decisions.

If stress alone were the causative agent in hypertension, then William should also have had high blood pressure. Yet he did not.

What Makes the Difference?

The difference in these two patients seemed to be explained by sociological factors. They were about the same age, but that's where the similarity ended. Unlike Diana, William had a very relaxed, outgoing personality. He told me that he had been brought up in an easygoing household; his family always had wine with their evening meals, and he remembered his father observing that "life is too short to be upset."

The surface physical differences between these two people were obvious. Diana was tall, thin, and tended to get flushed when she was animated. William was short, heavy-set, and olive-skinned. Diana was nervous and tense, whereas William was very relaxed. On that basis alone, one could have chosen the hypertensive person without much effort.

In this instance, the stress associated with the job seemed to be only a secondary factor. The primary factor was the difference in temperament and how each person dealt with stress. These two cases suggest that external stress alone does not cause hypertension.

War Is Hell—Sometimes

Some years ago, I served as a medical officer on the battleship *Wisconsin*. We were at that time involved in the Korean War and subject to all the stress that actual battle conditions produce. My battle station was in the ship's sick bay, a number of decks below the waterline.

During action, this area was sealed off so that if the ship was hit by a torpedo here, the remainder of the vessel would be unaffected. Therefore, the period of time that we were at battle stations was obviously stressful. Yet when I ran a series of studies to see what effect this situation had on the men, in no case did I find anyone with elevated blood pressure. The fact that the stress caused by this particular situation did not result in any increase in blood pressure would indicate that acute stress, when short-lived, is not the cause of hypertension.

On the other hand, some studies suggest that people subjected to constant stress may react differently. One, presented in the *American Medical News* of June 22, 1984, by free-lance writer William Hoffer, stated that in December 1978, Robert Rose, M.D., concluded a 5½-year study of air traffic controllers and found that high levels of hypertension were linked to periodic increases in air traffic. The study indicated that hypertension can be produced by acute stress if it is applied repeatedly for a long time.

The Role of Stress in Hypertension

What conclusions can one come to in regard to stress and the onset of hypertension? From the medical literature as well as my own experience I believe the following to be true:

1. Stress will cause hypertension in anyone who is stress-sensitive or who has a predetermined mechanism that responds to stress (or to repeated stress) by developing persistently high blood-pressure levels.

2. The condition of people who suffer from hypertension will be made worse when stress is superimposed. In the hypertensive person, stress will cause a rise in blood pressure that brings about the onset of complications sooner than would be the case if there were no stress.

3. People who are given to internally induced stress will develop high blood pressure even if no external stress exists.

From this, we can draw the following equations about the potential patterns of hypertension:

- Stress-sensitive individual + stress = hypertension
- Hypertensive person + stress = more severe hypertension and complications
- Internally stressed personality + routine life problems = hypertension

The General Adaptation Syndrome

By what mechanism does stress translate itself into hypertension? Researcher Hans Selye developed a physiological concept he recalled the "general adaptation syndrome," in which he said the body prepares to protect itself from danger by either "fight or flight"; that is, when confronted with stress, the body will prepare physiologically either to stand and fight or to run away.

To do so, the body makes changes in its internal system. One way is to increase the blood pressure within the arterial system to increase the supply of nutrients and oxygen to the muscles and the brain. Therefore, when confronted by stress, the body responds with a rise in blood pressure.

Eventually, if this is repeated often enough, the arteries attempt to protect themselves from the increased pressure on their walls and go into spasm—a tightening of the artery walls similar to tightening your fist. This narrowing brings about a further increase in pressure, causing more spasm. Imagine you are holding a soft hose in your hand. Now as you tighten your fist around the hose you are producing a situation similar to spasm in the artery. A vicious cycle develops: more pressure, more spasm, causing increased pressure.

How to Break the Stress-Hypertension Cycle

Any stress-producing situation will cause the body to respond in this hypertension-producing manner. The stress-sensitive blood system will eventually develop a constant rise in pressure or hypertension. To avoid this, one must break the cycle of stress-caused increased pressure. Fortunately, there are a number of ways to do this.

The first is rest. Rest is basic to the treatment and prevention of hypertension. It can be physical, emotional, or mental rest, and for most people it must be all three. To understand why rest is so basic to the therapy and prevention of hypertension, you should have some knowledge of the mechanism that produces the rise in pressure.

The vascular system is a series of pipes and tubes with areas that act as valves, causing an increase in resistance and thereby an increase in pressure. If you rest, you decrease the need for blood to pass through the system, and thus you decrease the demand for pressure. The more rest, the less need for blood flow, and the greater the drop in pressure.

It has been commonly observed that in hospital patients short periods of bed rest will reduce blood-pressure levels. True, the reduction is not very pronounced in older patients or in patients who have prolonged and severely elevated blood pressure, but it does hold true for the younger patients whose blood pressure still can be corrected. This observation clearly demonstrates the importance of simple physical rest. The greater the degree of rest, the better the response.

Ways to Relax at Work

You need not lie down to rest. You can rest by developing a system for relaxing. Consider your lunch hour. Divide the time: half for eating your lunch and half for relaxing. The relaxation can be as simple as sitting on a bench near the office and unwinding. Enjoy the day, or just watch the people go by. You can even relax at your desk by reading a novel. Whatever you do, put all your work problems and any other problems out of your mind.

Make a conscious effort to relax. Become aware of the sensation of actual relaxation in your muscles during this resting time. If you learn to relax, you will help decrease the tension in your system, which in turn will help lower blood-pressure levels.

Start doing this relaxation process for a few minutes at first, then increase the time to ten minutes, then longer. Once you have learned to relax totally, you should increase the frequency of these relaxation periods. On weekends, when you are not working, set aside a half hour after each meal for this positive relaxation procedure.

Ways to Relax at Home

This system of resting should not be limited to the workday. Sleep is the most basic rest of all, and it is important to use the period of time before going to bed to establish a rest pattern. "Home hydrotherapy" is an ideal way to start. Get into a bathtub filled with warm (not hot) water, and soak for fifteen minutes. Let your muscles relax; if you have been on your feet all day, gently massage your leg muscles to help them relax.

When you get into bed, stretch out full length and get into a comfortable position. Then, concentrating on nothing but your body, start with your head and work downward, relaxing each group of muscles as you progress. As you move down your body, relax your upper arm muscles, then your forearms, then your hands, your thigh muscles, your leg muscles, and eventually your feet.

During this process, you must work on your mind as well as your body. Clear your mind of any stressful thoughts. In fact, if you think of something very pleasant, you will discover that it helps you to relax. You might find music a helpful adjunct to this relaxation technique, but it should be soft music, not anything distracting.

Many people have no problem falling asleep but find they wake up after a few hours and are not able to get back to sleep. Fortunately, one need not actually sleep to obtain the benefits of rest. Simply stay in bed and either turn on the radio and listen to some music, or just lie there relaxing your muscles. In either case, you will continue to benefit from the rest even though you are not asleep.

Do a Little Each Day

There are many other ways to program rest periods into your life. Using a rocking chair for a ten-minute period each day will help give you the kind of relaxation you need. However, relaxation exercises are only part of the relaxation method.

Hobbies offer a wonderful approach to relaxation. Many people find painting or drawing or playing a musical instrument excellent ways to unwind. These artistic endeavors need have no other goal than simple enjoyment. Other people find activities like bird-watching a good means of relaxation. The potential avenues of relaxation are numerous. Don't take a passive approach to the problem but rather make positive steps toward developing this means of self-help. It takes only a little time and effort to determine what you like and how you can go about meeting your relaxation requirements.

How to Combat Mental Stress

Next, let's consider the various aspects of mentally produced stress. How can you develop a method for coping with mental stress? First you must develop the right mental attitude. Bear in mind that no matter how hard you work, nor how tense you let yourself become, you can't take it with you.

In "Elegy Written in a Country Churchyard," the poet Thomas Gray said: "The paths of glory lead but to the grave." For me, this single line has served as a constant reminder of the shortness of life and the end result of all our human strivings. It is something that I have kept in my mind's eye over the years, and it has become my mantra for relaxing when I find I am driving myself too hard.

Probably you, too, have some "direction line" that can restore your sense of perspective. You might even want to make it into a sign that you can keep in front of you as a reminder; even if you don't, you can try to keep it in the forefront of your mind at all times.

The Value of Meditation

I have been asked by patients about the value of various types of rest therapy and meditation. My advice is that rest is rest no matter what the form. If meditation enables you to maintain a restful state, then by all means use it as a helpful adjunct. The important point to remember is that rest is the key to therapy. The route by which it is attained is immaterial.

If you already have high blood pressure, there is a self-help technique you should know about. First, learn how to take and record your blood pressure. Next, schedule a program of rest at any time you wish during the day or in the evening. You select the time that you are going to rest, and before you start, check your blood pressure; check it again after the rest period is over.

In both instances, be sure to check it in the same manner. If, for example, you were sitting in a chair when you took your blood pressure before your rest, you should be in this position when you take it after resting. By keeping track of your pressure before and after, you can actually see how helpful these rest periods are for you.

Continue to concentrate on relaxing and on thinking relaxing thoughts. Try increasing your rest periods to see if that helps control your blood pressure. You will do well to give this self-help blood-pressure feedback therapy a try. It can do you no harm, and it may prove very helpful.

14

Biofeedback: A Relaxation Technique for Hypertension

Biofeedback is based on the concept that a person can learn to control physiological reactions such as muscle tension by controlling the reflex within the body that governs that action. Thus you can deliberately "feed back" into your system orders that will change reflex patterns to ones that are less stressful and healthier for you. Biofeedback has been demonstrated to slow the heart rate and reduce the blood pressure. Since hypertension is often a stress-related condition, biofeedback control of stress may well have value in the treatment of this disorder.

Biofeedback techniques use electronic equipment to identify the various electrical patterns that are produced within the body as a result of muscle contractions, heartbeat, and brain waves. It presents these normally silent reflex patterns as light patterns and sounds. As the electrical pattern within the body increases, the sound gets louder, and as the electrical pattern decreases, the sound, too, decreases. The person undergoing biofeedback tries to learn to control body function by creating changes in the light patterns or sounds. This control of sound and light, and thereby body function, usually is best attained by learning total relaxation.

Proponents of biofeedback have found it useful in treating a variety of stress-related conditions, including migraine and tension headaches, various gastrointestinal disorders (such as colitis and ulcers), asthma, insomnia, Raynaud's syndrome, menstrual pain, muscle spasm and pain, learning disabilities, hyperactivity, and last but not least, essential hypertension. It also has been used to alleviate hyperventilation as well as in rehabilitation following strokes, heart attacks, and various other injuries.

Physiological Feedback

Feedback is a familiar term in medicine. It is used to describe the body mechanism that keeps our internal environment stable within very fixed limits to ensure survival. One example is body temperature, which varies only a few degrees at any time in response to outside stimuli. You can best understand how this works if you compare body-temperature regulation to the heat and air-conditioning systems in a large building. When the outside temperature rises, the air conditioning goes on. When the temperature falls, the heat goes on. The thermostat that regulates the temperature in the building controlling the heat and air conditioning is really a feedback system that responds to temperature changes.

The respiratory tract offers another example of a feedback system within the body. When too much carbon dioxide builds up in the body, internal sensors send this knowledge to the brain, which informs the lungs to work a little faster and to breathe a little deeper to get the carbon dioxide out of the body. When too much is removed, the sensors inform the brain, and it slows the lungs so that less carbon dioxide is pushed out of the body. The system is kept in balance in this way. Of course, it is all done automatically; we are unaware that it is taking place, and we have no willful control over it.

Electronic Feedback

In the electronic feedback system used in biofeedback therapy, an attempt is made to understand the changes within the body and to control them willfully. Certain instruments are basic to biofeedback methodology; the electronic equipment commonly used to identify and study various body activities includes electromyographs, electroencephalographs, blood-pressure and heart-rate recorders, respiratory rate recorders, and dermographs.

The first of these, the *electromyograph* (EMG), is widely used in biofeedback training. It is an electrosensory recording system that picks up the minute electrical signals emitted by the muscles as they contract. An electrode or sensor is used to absorb the signal and magnify it so it can be seen on a screen, and this in turn can be presented in the form of popping sounds. The greater the degree of activity within the

155

muscle, the more sound is produced. In this fashion information is fed back to the individual so he or she can try to learn to control the degree of muscular activity. Initially, to learn the variables of control, patients tighten their muscles and move them. Later they work on relaxing these muscles.

EMG has been used as a tool in the treatment and management of stress. The idea is that if you can learn to relax your muscles, you can learn to control overall stress, and this can be facilitated by biofeedback.

How Biofeedback Works

An example of how this relaxation training works is given in the following excerpt from *From the Inside Out: A Self-Teaching and Laboratory Manual for Biofeedback* by Erik Peper and Elizabeth Ann Williams.

> Get in a comfortable position. Minimally tighten your right fist so that you feel only the smallest amount of tension. Hold it at this level. Be sure you continue to breathe.... Now let go and relax.... Observe the difference in feeling between the right and left arm and fist. Now minimally tighten your left fist. Hold this level so that you just feel the tightening.... Let go and relax. Let the relaxation spread through the arms and the rest of the body....

Following this technique, you can progress to actual visualization of your inner tension using the EMG. The object is first to identify tension and then to learn to relax your muscles so you can control the internal stress in your body.

Does It Really Work?

Does biofeedback work in cases of stress-related problems? Its proponents believe it is of value for any mental or physical symptoms with stress-related components. To date, critical evaluation of this concept is extremely difficult to produce. It is so vast a field and so without control studies that a true statistical evaluation is not possible. Obviously certain people in given situations would be greatly aided by the use of any relaxation technique. I can think of certain patients who are characteristic type A personalities—tense, driven to accomplish, and very uptight. For such persons, I believe that biofeedback therapy could be of definite value.

The typical case often cited in biofeedback literature involves a woman with tension headaches, who obtains substantial or total relief by learning to control the muscle tensions of her body, particularly those in the areas about the head. Clinically, however, cases like this are extremely difficult to evaluate.

The Brain-Wave Machine

Another instrument used in biofeedback, although its use is much more controversial than that of the EMG, is the *electroencephalograph* (EEG). The electroencephalograph, often referred to as the brain-wave machine because it records in graphic tracings the minute electrical waves produced by the brain cells as a result of their physiological functioning, is widely used in medical practice as a diagnostic tool. It can identify abnormal wave patterns associated with brain diseases such as epilepsy, tumors, and abscesses. It is of extreme diagnostic value in patients who have suffered convulsions, bouts of unconsciousness, or fainting spells. The waves are received by an electrode or sensor placed on the scalp and are magnified before being printed out in patterns on a moving tape. These wave patterns were first described in 1929 by the German physiologist Hans Berger, who named them alpha waves, beta waves, and delta waves, after letters of the Greek alphabet.

Alpha Waves

The wave pattern that is of special interest in biofeedback is the alpha wave. These waves are somewhat more specific than the other wave forms, being slow, rhythmic, and occurring in cycles that average about ten per second. For this reason, some EEG machines are specifically designed for use in biofeedback to record only these waves. Alpha waves are of particular importance because they are believed to be associated with a mental state that is alert but relaxed. The concept underlying biofeedback is directed toward reducing both internal and external stress, and the alpha waves are the measure of the state of relaxation that must be attained to find relief from systemic stress.

However, this relationship is not as simple as it might seem. There are factors that are not stress-related that can interfere with the alpha waves. Moreover, some claim that the alpha waves are easily altered and can even be increased when the subject's eyes are open rather than closed.

Using the Skin

Other instruments employed in biofeedback studies use the skin. One is a temperature gauge or *thermistor*, which measures the skin temperature; another is the *electrodermograph*, an instrument that measures changes in the electrical resistance of the skin.

The use of the thermistor to measure skin temperature in biofeedback therapy is based on the temperature of the skin being influenced by the autonomic nervous system. A breakdown in this system is believed to be responsible for causing a disorder called Raynaud's disease, as well as other diseases in which there is an inadequate supply of blood to the extremities. Presumably, if a patient with Raynaud's disease could learn via biofeedback to increase the skin temperature, he or she could increase the blood flow to the affected extremity, thereby controlling the disease process; however, to date, attempts to do this have not been very successful.

Biofeedback and Hypertension

Exactly what value does biofeedback have in the treatment of hypertension? The answer is not simple. Biofeedback has had a very checkered career. At its onset it was quickly seized by faddists and nonscientific workers who felt it would answer many problems that in fact it cannot. Certainly it is very appealing to think that you can learn to control the internal environment of your body and change unwanted reflex actions. Unfortunately, this has not proved true generally, although there are various areas in which biofeedback has produced excellent results, among them rehabilitation work on muscles, gait, muscle balance, and muscular reeducation.

In some people with hypertension, stress control via biofeedback is possible, but it would depend on the specific person. Hypertension has innummerable causes, and the disorder in a given patient may result from more than one cause. However, there is reason to believe that in patients in whom hypertension is triggered by stress alone, that factor often can be influenced by biofeedback.

Jan's Case

Jan began to have increasingly severe headaches about the time she was thirty, and when they began interfering with her demanding job, she sought medical advice. After a series of tests it was found that she had essential hypertension, which was causing the headaches. When she described her job, her physician suggested she try to find ways to alleviate the tension it caused her. On the advice of a friend, she tried biofeedback, and in her case the results were very gratifying. When she was away from work, she learned to relax by leaving her office problems in the office, where they belonged. Daily biofeedback exercises helped lower her blood pressure and bring relief from the headaches. In her case, this nonmedicinal therapy was all that was needed.

Learning to Monitor Blood Pressure

In one study conducted by D. A. Kristt and B. T. Engel, an attempt was made to teach people to control their blood pressure via biofeedback. A blood-pressure device was used so that each person could monitor his or her pressure. They were instructed to try to raise their pressure when a green light went on and to try to reduce it when a red light went on; when they were successful, a yellow light went on. Using this method, five patients were able to lower their systolic pressure from an average of 141mm Hg at home to an average of 125mm Hg at home while using methods they had learned in the laboratory. Although repeated attempts to reproduce this were unsuccessful, the conclusion was that biofeedback can temporarily lower blood pressure in patients with mild hypertension.

The Medical View of Biofeedback

A study group of the American College of Physicians evaluated the use of biofeedback in the treatment of hypertension and came to the following conclusions:

- Biofeedback cannot be recommended as first-line treatment for essential hypertension. It is suggested that the initial nondrug approach to the problem should be life-style counseling in such areas as weight reduction, regular exercise, reduction of salt intake, and discontinuance of smoking. (Interestingly, this group failed to mention a reduction in alcohol intake.)

- Biofeedback may be a useful adjunct in reducing medication requirements for patients with mild hypertension or for those who suffer adverse reactions to medication. As is the case with medication or other antihypertensive therapies, use of biofeedback requires careful monitoring of blood pressure. To date, studies indicate that biofeedback is no more effective than other relaxation therapies, such as yoga, meditation, and various self-relaxation techniques.

The report does note that results of studies using biofeedback for persons with mild to moderate essential hypertension (90 to 104mm Hg diastolic; 105 to 114mm Hg diastolic) suggest that some individuals can achieve moderate decreases in blood pressure (an average decrease of 8mm Hg systolic and 6mm Hg diastolic). The decreases in systolic blood pressure are greater than those obtained in diastolic. In general, these decreases are small and the duration of effects highly variable within given population groups, suggesting that certain people are more likely to benefit from this treatment than others.

The report recommends further randomized controlled trials with extended pretreatment base lines and long-term follow-up, including extensive monitoring of daily blood-pressure levels, to define better the degree and duration of effects with biofeedback. It points out that numerous issues about the method of treatment should be resolved, and in particular, an attempt should be made to determine which patients would be most likely to benefit from this and other non-medicinal treatments.

My Own Impression

My impression after reading this report is that its authors think there is value in the therapy but don't quite know how to evaluate the findings. Medical practice uses many varieties of therapy that aid only a fraction of the people being treated. If we knew at the start how to select those people who would benefit, our problems would be solved, but we don't. Therefore, the best approach is to try this therapy and then evaluate the results on a patient-by-patient basis. If the results are helpful, excellent. If they are not, the patient suffers no ill effects.

From my personal experience with this type of therapy, I am convinced that the ability to learn to relax is a very positive result, even if the drop in blood pressure is only slight. Note that the report says that in persons with mild to moderate essential hypertension the blood pressure dropped an average of 8mm Hg systolic and 6mm Hg diastolic; certainly these are excellent results. Obviously, had there been any evidence that blood pressure rose during biofeedback treatment, it should not be used; however, that was not the case.

In considering the value of biofeedback training in controlling hypertension, the diversity of causative factors must always be considered. There is a place for biofeedback in the treatment of hypertension. At present the clinical evidence is still in its infancy, but I believe the future will show that this therapy is a worthwhile adjunct. Readers who wish to have further information about biofeedback should turn to the Appendix, where various centers are listed.

15 ≈

How Exercise Combats Hypertension

We are coming more and more to recognize the value of regular exercise in combating a wide variety of diseases and disorders. Our sedentary life-style is as conducive to poor health as is our sugar-laden, high-fat diet. This appears to be as true for hypertension as for any other physical disorder.

The value of properly selected exercises in hypertensives cannot be disputed. In a study of 17,944 middle-aged civil service workers, the hypertensives in the group who were placed on a program of sports or exercise fared far better than the hypertensives who remained sedentary.

A number of studies have been conducted to evaluate the effect of exercise on blood pressure in men of various ages and with different pre-exercise (resting) blood-pressure levels. How does the effect of exercise in the person with normal blood pressure compare with changes in the hypertensive one?

In one study, involving forty-two men whose average age was forty and who had normal blood pressure, the resting diastolic blood-pressure levels after two months of strenuous exercise were below those at the beginning of the test. In a group of older men (average age, seventy) who were normotensive (that is, having blood pressure readings within the normal range) to start, both the diastolic and systolic pressure came down after six weeks of exercise. In another study, the diastolic pressure of a group of men, normotensive at the start, dropped 6mm Hg after six months of exercise; in a similar group, who were hypertensive to start, the diastolic pressure was down 12mm Hg after six months of exercise. The effect of selected exercise on the blood pressure of these hypertensive men was even more dramatic than in the normotensive men.

Exercise as a Preventive Measure

Is there any way to predict who will develop hypertension? Two excellent long-term studies were undertaken to try to make this determination: the University of Pennsylvania study and the Harvard study. The Pennsylvania study included 7,685 men under age thirty who had attended the school between 1931 and 1940. The cutoff year for the study was 1962. These men, all of whom were normotensive at the start of the study, were followed until 1962 (a follow-up of twenty-two to thirty-one years) and studied to analyze the effect on their lives of these four factors: participation in sports; body volume (weight); blood pressure at the start of the study; and the genetic factor—elevated blood pressure in their parents.

In the Pennsylvania study, 9 percent of those followed for twenty-two to thirty-one years developed elevated blood pressure. They ranged in age from twenty to sixty. Although a finding of 9 percent seems quite high, it is not at all out of line when you consider that there are an estimated 15 million Americans with hypertension today.

Of those men who had never participated in any kind of sports, 13.9 percent had high blood pressure, as opposed to a rate of 8.2 percent for those who engaged in some type of sports—an indication that exercise reduces the chance of developing hypertension. This finding has been confirmed in various other studies as well.

Hypertension was present in 10 percent of the men who were overweight, as opposed to only 7.9 percent in those who were not, an indication that excess weight contributes to hypertension. And men with elevated blood pressure early in the study tended to have continued increases in pressure as time went by. Those men whose parents had high blood pressure tended to develop it, too.

These last two findings also were confirmed by the results of the Harvard study, which included 15,000 men who attended the school and were followed for six to ten years thereafter. This study found that gaining weight increased the risk of hypertension and confirmed that hypertension occurred less often in those men who took part in vigorous sports than it did in sedentary men. The worst combination was lack of activity coupled with excess weight. Physical activity plays a major role in keeping pressure down. Simply keeping your weight down is not enough; you must be active, too.

Why Exercise Is Important to Physical Well-Being

First of all, exercise does two very essential things for the body: It burns up energy, and it builds muscles. If we did not burn up energy, all the food we eat would automatically turn to fat. Indeed, as we get older and become less active, an energy imbalance develops: Too many calories in, not enough out. The result is new fat, increased weight, and increased potential for high blood pressure. Adequate physical exercise brings a decrease in weight, a decrease in blood pressure, and a decrease in essential hypertension.

Although most discussions of exercise stress the physical changes and benefits that can be derived, I believe the most important advantage is the feeling of well-being. One has only to start on a physical-fitness program to experience the sense of exhilaration that ensues. This "good" feeling is now believed to result from an increase in the opioid-peptides, which are a kind of naturally occurring narcotic in the body. Certainly, if essential hypertension has as its basis an element of stress, then an increase in the opioid-peptides that contribute to a feeling of well-being can only lead to a sense of ease that is beneficial in lessening hypertension.

Feeling Well and Looking Good

As a secondary benefit, a feeling of well-being also can aid in keeping food intake down. It is far easier to watch calories when you are feeling good about yourself than when you are depressed, as the case of Susan,

167

a twenty-one-year-old patient of mine, bears out. Susan had a weight problem, and numerous attempts to diet met with only temporary success. The few pounds she lost when she started to diet were quickly put back on as soon as she resumed her normal routines. She found the answer to her weight problem by joining an exercise group at the local Y. She explained that the daily exercises and swim made her feel "really good," and she noted that when she got home after exercising she felt no need to run to the refrigerator and "just pack it in." For her, the good feeling solved her desire to overeat. She has remained on this program for more than a year, with excellent results.

Types of Exercise

Basically there are three main types of exercise: isotonic or aerobic, isometric, and isokinetic. *Isotonic* or *aerobic exercise* involves the repeated and constant use of the large muscles of the body; this produces a response from the cardiovascular system by calling forth a marked increase in blood flow to the muscles to meet their needs for oxygen and the removal of metabolic wastes. Walking, jogging, swimming, and cycling are examples of this kind of exercise.

Weight lifting is an example of an *isometric exercise*. Although it produces massive enlargement of the muscles (witness those enormous men on television during the Olympics straining to lift hundreds of pounds), it is not of much value to the cardiovascular system. Furthermore, not only is it inadvisable to use these exercises if you have high blood pressure, it may in fact be dangerous.

Isokinetic exercise is comparatively new; it develops

muscular strength by means of specially designed exercise equipment such as rowing machines or exercise bicycles. This type of exercise depends on the presence of a resistance equal to the force applied by the person doing the exercise.

How Does Exercise Alter Blood Pressure?

Any type of exercise causes an immediate rise in blood pressure, but it is short-term, lasting only as long as the exercise. The rise in blood pressure follows a physiological pattern, which explains why some exercises are good for you and others are dangerous. When you exercise, the rise in blood pressure can be as high as 80mm Hg or as low as 20mm Hg, depending on the body's response to stress resulting from the demand for energy. The nervous system charges up all the body systems and, in so doing, increases the central body blood pressure. This is done by a special branch of the nervous system, the sympathetic branch, which prepares the body for increased efforts. When you use a muscle for work or exercise, it calls for an increase in blood flow by opening numerous blood vessels. This draws blood from the central system, decreasing the pressure in direct proportion to the amount of pressure accepted by the newly opened blood vessels.

If you use only a few muscles, the decrease in central pressure is slight, and the body pressure can rise quite high. When you use large numbers of muscles, as in swimming, cross-country skiing, or jogging, the newly opened vessels draw off a large volume of blood, reducing the central level. Exercises that use large numbers of muscles are best for the person with

169

essential hypertension. The pressure rises only a little, and the danger of a blood-vessel rupture is slight.

When Isn't Exercise Advisable?

People with hypertension secondary to tumors of the adrenal gland, diseases of the thyroid gland, kidney disease, any disease that occurs within the brain, or any disease of the main artery of the body, the aorta, should refrain from exercise that may elevate the blood pressure. Why is this so? What might happen under such circumstances? For one thing, increased pressure can sorely test the strength of the arterial walls. If there are areas of weakness, increased pressure can cause the walls to rupture, which is what happens when someone has an aneurysm.

Some studies suggest that exercise is not always beneficial even in those with essential hypertension. I mention them to give a balanced view, although I believe, as a result of my experience, that exercise is of great value to this group.

An often-cited study* involved a group of hypertensive children whose resting blood pressures were high. After exercise, their pressures went up beyond the elevation typically found in normotensive children, a predictable finding given the fact that the blood vessels of these children were already tight, a situation the stress of exercise aggravated. All the research on hypertension, including the Pennsylvania and Harvard studies, indicates that when the pressure is high to start, it tends to get worse. However, exercise of the correct

*James, F. W., "Effects of Physical Stress on Adolescents," *Post Grad. Med.*, 56:53, 1974. Cited in *Diet and Exercise: Synergism in Health Maintenance*, AMA Publication, 1982.

type, done under controlled conditions, will decrease the degree of elevation.

The key to exercise as a means of preventing and helping control high blood pressure depends entirely on the correct use of this therapy. The exercises should not be too taxing; they should be increased on a progressive basis and done regularly so there is no sudden or undue strain. Overexertion or too great stress at any one time should always be avoided.

How to Determine If an Exercise Program Is Safe for You

A good start, prior to any exercise program, is compilation of a careful medical history as well as a doctor's physical examination, including various blood tests and urine analyses. If your history reveals any potential illnesses or if your physical exam reveals any abnormalities, they should be evaluated and/or corrected before you start.

A Program for the No-Exercise Exerciser

The no-exercise exerciser is someone who has not exercised at all in the past. If you fit this description, start by selecting a routine you can do when you get out of bed in the morning. Once you start, make it a rule that you will do this exercise daily, and don't skip a day. When you get into a pattern of regular exercise you will find it becomes increasingly easier to continue. The beauty of simple exercises is that they require no equipment and not very much room.

Start with as many of the following simple routines as you can comfortably do:

1. *Stretch both arms outward* and gently rotate them, first forward and then backward, in small circles. Start with three each way, each day, and increase the number during the week, always at least maintaining the previous day's number.

2. *Raise your arms over your head* and stretch them as far forward and as far backward as you can before lowering them. Breathe deeply with each stretching action. Fill your lungs as you raise your arms, and slowly let the air out as you lower them. (Do not do this in too quick succession, since it is possible to hyperventilate, which can cause you to become dizzy.)

3. *Next, rotate your head* in a complete circle. Stretch your neck muscles by pushing your chin down on your chest. Next, stretch your head back as far as you can; then stretch it to one side and then to the other.

4. *Try to touch your toes.* Do so gently; do not force yourself too far, for it is possible to injure the ligaments in your knees if you press too hard. If you cannot get down all the way, spread your legs farther apart until you can touch the floor.

5. *Next, place your hands on your shoulders* and turn the palms upward. Now raise both hands as if you were lifting something over your head. Stretch all the way up. Now slowly

lower your hands in the same position in which you raised them. Do this three times to start. You will feel the tension in the arm muscles that you used for this exercise, which normally are not used very often. You can do this exercise with your head back and then with your head forward.

6. *Next bring one knee up* so you are standing on one foot. Pull the knee upward with your hands. Then lower the leg and do the same thing with the other knee. Next, extend each leg as far back and then as far forward as you can. Swing each leg outward and hold it in that position for a while, the longer the better.

7. *If you are having trouble with your abdominal muscles,* here are two good exercises: The first helps identify the muscles that need added tone; the second, which is more strenuous, will tighten these muscles.

Draw your stomach muscles in and, at the same time, press your fingertips deeply into the muscles on each side of your abdomen. Apply pressure to these muscles through your fingertips, and then push outward against your fingers. Tighten these muscles, then loosen them and press hard against your fingertips. This exercise is twofold, as it helps you learn to control these muscles and also helps to strengthen them.

The next exercise—sit-ups—may be difficult to do at first, but if you work at it regularly you will find that eventually it is painless. As always, start slowly and increase the number each day. Lie flat on your back and hook your feet under a bed, couch, or chest to stabilize them. Put your hands behind your head and slowly lift your head, bringing your elbows to touch your knees. Then lower yourself back down. This is an excellent exercise if done slowly over a period of time.

Routines for the Occasional Exerciser

The occasional exerciser is someone who cannot bring himself or herself to do strenuous daily exercises but who does want to do *some* exercise regularly. If this sounds like you, try to set up a three-times-a-week schedule. For example, set aside time on Tuesday, Thursday, and Saturday for your workout.

Here is an easy exercise for the city dweller who may find such typical occasional exercise such as cycling, golf, or hiking hard to do. If you live in an apartment house, start your exercise by walking up one flight of stairs once a day. Then increase it to two times a day. Once you are used to the one-flight routine, try two flights and continue two flights a day, progressing to two flights twice a day. Then move on to three flights.

Since I live on the third floor, I have accustomed myself to the three-flight program. Walking up steps is one of the simplest means of exercise. To date, the best use I've seen made of this method is by a colleague of mine, who walks up twelve flights of stairs to the operating room every morning, an exercise he has come to find essential.

A home rowing machine is an excellent aid to encourage exercise. They are available in many department stores and in most athletic stores as well in various sales catalogs. They are unique in that there is no other exercise equipment I know of that has one use all the muscles, including both arms and legs, this machine requires. The exercise itself is very pleasant, which is an inducement to doing it routinely.

Exercises for the Moderate Daily Exerciser

The moderate daily exerciser should start by buying an exercise bicycle (or a rowing machine) for home use. There are many models to choose from. Select one that has a device for controlling the degree of resistance against which you must pedal. Start with a low degree of resistance and slowly increase it as you progressively increase the amount of time you spend pedaling.

One simple exercise that requires no equipment is running in place. You can start by running for two minutes and then increase the time for as long as it feels comfortable. And, of course, you can institute a daily exercise routine using any or all of the exercises on the preceding pages.

Swimming is excellent exercise. Water provides the same kind of resistance that the exercise bicycle does. To increase the amount of exercise, simply increase the number of laps you swim if you are using a pool, and then increase the speed at which you do the distance.

Jogging has become very popular in recent years. However, it should be done with an element of temperance. Carried past a certain point, jogging does not produce commensurate value and can lead to foot and knee problems. I have seen many joggers increase the distance they jog by miles, but I am not sure this does not eventually encounter the law of diminishing returns.

Outdoor cycling is an excellent and ever-popular form of exercise. Some of the new cycles are extremely light in weight, so that riding is comfortable and pleasant. During the gasoline shortage a few years ago, I decided to go to the hospital by bicycle. At first it seemed a bit taxing, but after a while I came to like it so much that now it is the way I prefer to travel in nice weather. In many cities, cycle clubs have one-day or even longer trips. You may find the group activity a help in getting committed to your exercise regimen.

Cross-country skiing is another excellent means of exercise because it involves muscles that are seldom used. It requires far less technical skill than downhill skiing, and you can move along as fast or as slowly as you wish, so that it is both very relaxed and stimulating. As a final plus, the skis are much cheaper than downhill equipment, and you don't need a lift ticket. In fact, all you need is an open field or a city park and some snow.

The Dedicated Exerciser

The dedicated exerciser is the person who works at physical fitness constantly. I have had the experience of living with this type of individual—my eldest son, who from early childhood was self-motivated to exercise daily. You need only ask him to show how many push-ups he can do and he will gladly do a hundred. He lifts weights, and every morning he gets up and runs a mile or two. He has a built-in desire, one I do not believe can be forced in any way. However, I do think you can encourage someone to follow a course of moderate exercise, and as a doctor that is what I try to do, both as a personal goal and as a recommendation to my patients and friends.

Health Clubs

If you like exercise and recognize the benefits, consider joining a health club. Most cities have these clubs, which have excellent facilities and good instructors. You will probably find the money well spent. In fact, I have spoken with many people who say that the club helped them get on an exercise program and stay on it. One patient told me that she is committed to exercise because she paid for the club membership and feels it a waste if she does not attend.

Whatever your reason for exercising, doing it is what counts.

IV

HYPERTENSION DRUGS

~~~~~~

Everything you need to know about what they are, how they can help, and their side effects and problems.

16 〰

A Word on Antihypertensive Drugs and When to Use Them

Prior to 1950, a diagnosis of hypertension was truly a death sentence. The rice diet helped some people but it often wasn't enough. What might begin with something as simple as a headache—the first symptom of the markedly elevated blood pressure discovered later in the doctor's office—could progress until the patient had a stroke or heart attack. Some people might suffer severe nosebleeds when their pressure was high—a symptom of the body's desperate attempt to decrease mounting pressure by decreasing the volume of blood within the system. In those days, the only treatment to reduce the blood pressure consisted of a low-salt diet, bed rest, and possibly the use of phenobarbital—"sleeping pills." However, very little helped, and the situation generally worsened. The advent of specific antihypertensive drugs has changed this picture.

When Possible, Use Nondrug Therapy

However, the use of these medicines is not always the best choice in initiating treatment for hypertension, according to most authorities in the field. Dr. Norman K. Kaplan, professor of medicine at the University of Texas and author of a widely used medical textbook, *Clinical Hypertension*, advocates that, whenever possible, nondrug therapies such as sodium restriction, weight reduction, relaxation techniques, and exercise be used to lower the blood pressure before turning to the more risky use of medications. Nondrug therapy (good nutrition, weight control, stress control, alcohol and sodium restriction, no smoking, and exercise) is better than drugs in people with mild elevations of pressure or in those with a predisposition to hypertension, since these techniques are not only effective in reducing hypertension but also can curb its development. These drugless methods aid the general well-being of anyone following them, but they are not always enough. Let me stress again that you must work with your doctor to find the right treatment for you. If drugless methods do not lower your pressure enough, what are your choices?

Combined Treatment

In many cases, an intelligent blend of drugless methods with carefully selected medications is the best approach to the problem of hypertension. The value of medication for many patients cannot be questioned, and I would in no way suggest that one should avoid medication or stop taking it if it has been prescribed (never stop taking your medicine suddenly or without your doctor's knowledge). I would encourage any patient to incorporate nondrug therapies along with medication to obtain the best results.

Just How Valuable Is Medication?

The answer to that question is: very valuable indeed. The efficacy of treatment with drugs has been demonstrated in many studies. In one, conducted by the Veterans Administration, a group of seventy men who had diastolic blood pressure readings ranging from 115 to 129mm Hg were left untreated. Of this group, four died of cardiovascular disease and twenty-three had serious complications from hypertension. Another group, of seventy-three men with the same diastolic pressure readings, were treated with medication; none died of cardiovascular disease, and only two had serious complications.

In another study of men with diastolic blood pressure readings ranging from 90 to 114, nineteen who were untreated died of cardiovascular disease and fifty-seven had complications. In the treated group only eight died of cardiovascular disease and fourteen had complications.*

The value of medications in the treatment of hypertension has been established. Before antihypertensive medications were available, the degree and frequency of complications were far higher than they are now.

*Studies cited in Timothy N. Caris, M.D., *A Clinical Guide to Hypertension*. PSG Publishing Co., Littleton, MA, p. 71. Original in *AMA* 1967 and 1970.

Indications for Initiating Treatment

Despite the very clear indications that medications can be both life-saving and health-preserving, there is considerable controversy over the preferred methods and when such therapy should be started. Before we consider the problems of when to treat and how, let's examine those aspects of therapy about which there is no controversy. It is generally agreed that anyone with elevated blood pressure, no matter how mild, should be monitored. Blood-pressure levels should be checked regularly and, depending upon the degree of elevation, various tests, such as electrocardiograms, chest X rays, and blood and urine studies should be made. The frequency with which the blood pressure should be checked is determined by many factors, but the higher the readings, the more frequent the monitoring should be.

In some cases, the cause of high blood pressure can be determined; initially, in treating any patient with hypertension, the possibility of finding the cause and correcting it should always be considered. However, high blood pressure is often idiopathic—that is, the cause cannot be determined and/or corrected.

The need for observation and treatment is greater in younger patients (under puberty) with hypertension, because they have poor tolerance for this disorder and the likelihood that they will develop serious complications is far greater. Consequently, any young person with high blood pressure is at risk and needs treatment.

It is also agreed that treatment is indicated when the diastolic blood pressure exceeds 100 because complications are likely to occur with this level of diastolic pressure. For those patients whose pressure is below 100 diastolic but over 80 diastolic, several questions should be asked. Do they need treatment? If so, how much? When should it be started?

Treatment is clearly indicated for people with the following complicating risk factors:

- *High blood cholesterol.* People with high blood cholesterol levels face a greater risk of heart disease than do others. The relationship is very direct: The risk rises as the blood cholesterol level goes up. In fact, the level that for a long period of time was considered normal—250— now seems to be too high for the patients's good. The National Institutes of Health presented the following data on blood cholesterol levels:*

	Cholesterol Level Presents	
Age	Moderate Risk at Greater than	High Risk at Greater than
2–19	170	185
20–29	200	220
30–39	220	240
40 +	240	260

- *Smoking.* People who smoke face a higher risk of coronary disease than those who do not because smoking directly increases both systolic and diastolic blood pressure.

- *Diabetes.* Diabetes constitutes an increased risk both directly, as a disease that damages blood

---

*Abstracted from an article in *Transition*, May 1984.

vessels and thereby increases the dangers of various types of cardiovascular disease, and indirectly, as a disease that in itself requires careful medical monitoring.

- *Heredity.* A family history of complications due to hypertension is extremely significant. The presence of these complications within a family indicates a genetic weakness, and the statistics bear this out. Because of an inherent weakness, the complications of hypertension often occur in such people at lower levels of pressure than is the case with others.

- *Hypertension.* High blood pressure itself is a major risk factor in causing strokes, cerebrovascular disease, heart disease, kidney disease, and eye disease. Therefore, the presence of high blood pressure with a concomitant finding of any of these disease processes indicates that the need for blood-pressure control is both essential and urgent.

The Effects of Complications

What happens to patients who develop various complications? Complications may result in the loss of kidney function so that the kidneys are unable to clear the body of the waste products of metabolism. Eventually this leads to a disease process called uremia. When uremia occurs, an artificial kidney is required to maintain body function. The physician can test for the development of this disease by the blood urea nitrogen (BUN) test, which indicates the blood level of the waste products remaining within the body. Kidney damage is a very serious complication of high blood pressure, and the outcome can be fatal.

Damage to the heart is equally serious. Changes in the electrocardiogram may indicate that the heart is having difficulty pumping against increased pressure in the vascular system. As the need for more pressure develops, the heart muscles will start to enlarge and thicken, in much the same way that the muscles of a weight lifter thicken and increase in size as he works against heavier and heavier weights. Unfortunately, where the heart muscle is concerned, there is a point beyond which it cannot increase its size or strength, and when this happens, heart failure occurs. Heart failure is manifested by shortness of breath, weakness, fatigue, and collection of fluid within the legs, face, and elsewhere in the body. Eventually the heartbeat develops irregularities.

Among the eye complications that can occur is leakage of blood from minute blood vessels into the back of the eye. The physician can directly examine the back of the eye with an ophthalmoscope and visualize this leakage and the spasm of the blood vessels.

The presence of other diseases increases the danger of complications of hypertension and heightens the need for treatment. For example, gout can injure the blood vessels as well as the kidneys and the joints of the body; immediate treatment is essential.

Initiating Drug Therapy

Once the various criteria that determine the need for drug treatment are found to be present, what should be done?

First, it is important that the patient understand the

need to utilize the standard nondrug treatments: weight control, exercise, salt reduction, adequate nutritional intake, stress control, and rest. When medicines are given, careful medical monitoring is essential to determine the correct dosage and to spot any adverse reactions or side effects; the patients must be made aware that this monitoring is necessary and must agree to cooperate in the medical follow-up.

Diuretics

Drug therapy is based on a stepped-progression concept. This means just what the name suggests. The dosage and the number of medications given are increased progressively until the desired degree of blood-pressure control is attained. The medications that initially are most widely used belong to a group of chemicals known as the thiazide diuretics. These medicines increase the production of urine; when this happens, the body expels sodium and potassium as well as large volumes of water. These drugs also help the blood flow within the arteries. A decrease in the volume of blood and body fluids has the effect of lowering blood pressure. These drugs also work directly on the muscles of the arteries, helping them to relax and thus lowering the blood pressure.

Combating Potassium Loss

However, diuretics can have unpleasant side effects. Nausea, muscle cramps, loss of too much body fluids, loss of too much sodium or potassium, retention of body waste products, increased blood sugar (as with diabetes), and rash all can occur.

If you are using these medications, your doctor should carefully monitor their effects. The dosage must be increased or decreased, depending on your response. Your progress must be followed to be sure that in the process of reducing your body's sodium content, there has not been an unwanted loss of potassium, which passes out in the urine along with sodium. This loss of potassium can be corrected by increasing dietary potassium, which can easily be done by eating bananas and dried fruits or by drinking orange juice. Potassium supplements, in the form of pills or a liquid, also can be given to counteract the problem of potassium loss.

Yet another method of controlling potassium loss—and the one that is the most widely used—is to give a thiazide diuretic in combination with a diuretic that specifically helps retain potassium. The most commonly used medication of this type is Dyazide, an antihypertensive capsule that combines a thiazide diuretic with a potassium-conserving medication called triamterene. This agent increases the urinary output, removing fluid and sodium from the body, but retains potassium.

How successful is this drug in treating hypertension? Many studies indicate that 80 percent of patients with high blood pressure can be treated successfully with it. It is the simplest and least dangerous of the antihypertensive agents, causes the least imbalance in the physiology of the body, and has the fewest side effects.

The antihypertensive effect of diuretics can be offset by an intake of sodium. If the dietary sodium intake reaches a level of 15 to 20 g a day, it can offset the loss of sodium produced by the diuretic, making the diuretic ineffective. On the other hand, if the dietary sodium intake is reduced too sharply while these salt-losing diuretics are being taken, it is possible to produce too great a decrease in the sodium content of the body.

If the potassium loss becomes too great and there is inadequate replacement, signs of potassium insufficiency will occur, manifested by weakness, leg cramps, and a feeling of chronic fatigue. If this loss is allowed to progress, it will interfere with the normal contractions of the heart. To prevent this, blood tests should be run to determine the potassium levels, and correct action taken if necessary. In some cases the changes connected with severe potassium loss will appear on the electrocardiogram. The complexity of maintaining the proper potassium balance is yet another reason for constant medical observation when these drugs are used.

Step Therapy

In patients for whom simple thiazide diuretic medication does not control blood pressure, step therapy must be tried. In this type of therapy, stronger and stronger medicines are added progressively until the proper control is obtained. Increasing the drug strengthens its antihypertensive effect, producing changes in all levels of body function. Step therapy can take different forms, involving different combinations of drugs. One of the commonly used progressions is as follows:

- Step 1: administration of a thiazide diuretic
  If that does not work, add
- Step 2: propranolol hydrochloride or methyl-dopa or reserpine
  If unsuccessful, add
- Step 3: hydralazine hydrochloride
  If necessary, add or substitute
- Step 4: guanethidine sulfate

Side Effects Can Occur

As is often the case, effective results sometimes are accompanied by side effects. Some of the side effects produced by these potent drugs include:

- Kidney damage
- Increased blood calcium levels
- Loss of potassium
- Sensitivity to light
- Loss of blood cells
- Swelling of breasts
- Drowsiness
- Abnormal hair growth
- Loss of consciousness upon standing
- Insomnia
- Headache
- Loss of ability to ejaculate
- Loss of potency
- Heart palpitations
- Rashes
- Intestinal problems

If you are taking these drugs you should immediately notify your physician if any of these complications occurs.

A review of this list gives one pause, for the side effects are extensive and potentially serious. However, you must weigh the possible dangers of the medicine against the dangers of high blood pressure, and the choice must be made on the basis of a comparative evaluation of each. In the end, the complications of seriously elevated blood pressure are invariably more severe and life-threatening than are the side effects of this medication. For that reason, treatment is generally indicated despite the possible side effects.

To complete the picture of drug therapy for hypertension, one must acknowledge a vast array of medications under development, offering the potential for better control of hypertension with less danger. Many authorities now feel that one need no longer start with the thiazide diuretics, as was done in the past, but can use various other drugs instead. Time will, of course, answer that question. At present, progressive step therapy is the most widely used treatment and to date historically the most successful.

An Analysis of Some of the Drugs Commonly Used for Hypertension

In a recent survey, six of the ten most commonly prescribed drugs were antihypertensive and heart medications, which gives some indication of the vast number of people afflicted with these disorders. While it would be impossible to list every cardiac and hypertensive medication here, I will discuss some of the most commonly used ones and will outline what each does for you and what to watch out for if you are taking it.

As is the case with any medication, you must adhere carefully to the dosage program your physician has prescribed. If you do not, you will not get the maximum benefit from the medication and, indeed, may get poor results. Should you develop an untoward reaction to any medication, *always* discontinue it and call your doctor at once.

Dyazide, first on the list and the most widely used, already has been discussed but is presented again here because a new combination of its components has been placed on the market in the form of a medication called *Maxzide*. Unlike Dyazide, which has 25 mg of hydrochlorothiazide and 50 mg of triamterene, Maxzide contains 50 mg of hydrochlorothiazide and 75 mg of triamterene, and it is claimed that only one tablet a day is needed as compared with two a day for Dyazide. The hydrochlorothiazide pushes sodium and water out of the body, causing the loss of some potassium, an effect the triamterene helps to counteract.

If you compare these two drugs, you will find:

- 2 Dyazide = 50 mg hydrochlorothiazide + 100 mg triamterene
- 1 Maxzide = 50 mg hydrochlorothiazide + 75 mg triamterene

Since the only difference between the two is 25 mg of triamterene, the major value of the new drug would appear to be its one-a-day dosage.

The main reason for this new drug combination, which is so similar to the old one, is that the patent on Dyazide has run out, so that other companies may now produce and sell similar drugs, a situation that will shortly affect the makers of Inderal, Aldomet, and Minipress. The net result is that the price of all these drugs will come down.

HYPERTENSION DRUGS

Lasix (furosemide) is a widely used diuretic agent that acts on the kidneys, forcing them to excrete sodium and water. Increased urination usually starts one hour after taking the pill by mouth and reaches its maximal effect in two hours. Its total length of action is between six and eight hours. However, it is so potent that the dosage must be carefully controlled, since it is possible to lose so much sodium and water that dehydration and/or circulatory collapse may result. This is one of the reasons why it is so important that this drug be given under the close supervision of a physician and that the effects of the drug be monitored.

Because results of studies in animals show that this drug can cause abnormalities in the fetus, it should not be given to women who could become pregnant, unless their condition is so life-threatening that the drug is essential.

There are a great many other potential side effects associated with use of this drug; among them are skin rash, itching, blurring of vision, sudden loss of blood pressure upon standing, nausea, vomiting, diarrhea, loss of white cells in the blood, weakness, fatigue, and dizziness.

Slow-K, a 600-mg, sugar-coated potassium tablet, and *Polycitra*, a liquid, are two potassium supplements commonly given to people being treated with diuretics. As was mentioned before, a loss of too much potassium can bring on a variety of symptoms, and physicians try to prevent this by frequent testing of the blood to see how much potassium is present. The normal blood level is between 3.5 and 5 mEq/L. If the level is dropping, a potassium supplement is indicated. If this level is down, it can often be corrected simply by increasing the amount of potassium-rich foods in the daily diet, without having to resort to supplements. A list of these foods appears on pages 110–111.

Aldomet (methyldopa) is a unique antihypertensive agent; its exact method of action is not known, although it appears to have an antihormonal effect. Because it reduces blood pressure without interfering with kidney function, it is widely used.

The drop in blood pressure produced by this drug may be greater when one is standing or walking, which can result in a feeling of faintness or weakness. The drug also can cause dryness of the mouth, drowsiness, anemia, or fever. In the male it may cause impotence. While many of these symptoms can be corrected by changing the dosage, at times it is necessary to change to a different medication.

If you are placed on this drug, your doctor will check your liver function and white-cell count, particularly during the first six to eight weeks, as the drug can depress both. If you use Aldomet in combination with another antihypertensive agent, the effects of each will be increased, a possibility you should be aware of. Despite its side effects, this strong agent is very effective when needed.

Hygroton (chlorthalidone) is another diuretic that is similar to the diazide diuretics but has a different chemical makeup. It produces its antihypertensive action by blocking the reabsorption of sodium into the body, thus causing a loss of water. The advantages of this drug are: It is excreted unchanged in the urine and therefore does not build up within the body; and it can be taken once a day, which makes it easier for patients to use. It has a number of side effects and cannot be given to anyone with kidney disease, as it may cause complete shutdown of kidney function. Unless there is a great need for it, it should not be used by any woman who could be pregnant because it can cause injury to the fetus.

Lopressor (metoprolol), *Inderal* (propranolol), and *Corgard* (nadolol) are beta-blocking drugs. Although the exact mechanism of their action is not known, they do interfere with the part of the autonomic nervous system that influences the heart rate. They produce a decrease in the heart rate, a decrease in the amount of blood that is pushed out of the heart with each beat, a decrease in the output of the hormone renin, and a decrease in the tone of the arteries, whose tightness causes the hypertension.

These drugs can be used alone or with the previously described diuretics. Side effects include asthma; extreme slowing of the heart; and some nervous system problems such as insomnia, depression, and fatigue; they also can cause impotence in some men. Despite the possible side effects, these drugs are widely used, with excellent results.

Tenormin (atenolol), another of the beta blockers, shares their actions and side effects but has the advantage that it need be given only once a day, making it an easier drug to use from the patient's point of view.

Rauwolfia (reserpine) drugs are central-nervous-system depressants that have less of an antihypertensive effect than one would like but do produce a mild sedative effect and work well when combined with other antihypertensive agents, such as diuretics.

As a central-nervous-system depressant, rauwolfia should never be given to anyone with a history of mental depression because it may make that condition worse; in extreme cases it has led to suicide. It also can cause drug dependency, insomnia, loss of appetite, and impotence.

Procardia (nifedipine) is a new type of anti-anginal and anti-hypertensive medication called a calcium channel blocker. It stops calcium from entering cells, which sometimes occurs in the heart muscle and in the muscles of the arteries, thereby preventing them from functioning. It aids in the prevention of anginal pain by relaxing the coronary arteries, and it lowers the blood pressure by relieving the tension in the small arteries that causes hypertension. The drop in pressure usually is between 5 and 10mm Hg systolic, although it can be more. Because the drug is so powerful, the side effects are many and varied. There can be a drop in blood pressure beyond what might be considered safe. Retention of water, called edema, also can result from the use of this drug. There are numerous other potential side effects, including changes in the chemistry of the liver, dizziness, giddiness, flushing and sensation of heat, headache, weakness, nausea, heartburn, muscle cramps, nervousness, palpitation, and sore throat. Because this drug can be life-saving, the dangers of its use are amply compensated by its value in certain situations.

Apresoline (hydralazine) and *Minipress* (prazosin) are drugs that dilate the arteries. They cause vasodilation and decrease the blood pressure by releasing the tension produced in the arteries. They are excellent antihypertensive agents because they act in a very physiological manner: They ease the passage of blood by decreasing the degree of blockage in the arteries. They, too, have side effects, including headaches, palpitations, and rapid heartbeat. The sudden drop in blood pressure that can occur when the user stands up (called orthostatic hypotension) poses a possible danger when taking these medications.

Capoten (captopril) is a unique antihypertensive

medication that works by blocking the normal physiological mechanism that regulates the blood pressure. When the blood pressure within the body drops (or when there is a blockage in the artery that supplies the kidneys), the blood flow into the kidneys is decreased. The body is so sensitive to this problem that it will immediately try to increase the blood flow by producing a rise in pressure in an attempt to protect the kidneys, which are essential to survival. It does so by activating the kidneys to produce an enzyme called renin, which starts a chain of chemical changes to raise the blood pressure.

The enzyme renin works on another chemical in the blood called angiotensinogen, turning it into a substance called angiotensin 1. Because this is not a strong enough hypertensive agent, the body converts it by means of a "converting enzyme" into angiotensin 2. Angiotensin 2 is an extremely powerful blood-pressure stimulant that tightens up the arteries and causes a rapid rise in pressure due to the increased resistance to the flow of blood. (It also increases pressure by causing the production of a hormone called aldosterone, which forces the kidneys to work in such a way that sodium and water are retained, both of which raise the blood pressure.)

The control of blood pressure by means of the renin system can be diagramed as follows:

Decrease of blood pressure = decrease in blood
                                      going into the
                                      kidneys
Kidneys release renin → works on angiotensino-
                                      gen → forms angioten-
                                      sin 1

Angiotensin 1 (weak material) + converting
enzyme
produces
Angiotensin 2 (strong tensor agent)
causes
Rise in blood pressure
More blood is forced into the kidneys / Body
returns to balance

These are all normal physiological steps in blood-pressure control.

Capoten works by blocking the converting enzyme from changing angiotensin 1 into angiotensin 2. Its potency is demonstrated by the fact that it can interfere so effectively with a basic body function. Like all medications that are strong and often life-saving, Capoten also carries a list of serious complications. When it is used with other antihypertensive agents, it can cause such a pronounced drop in blood pressure that hypotension and even shock may result. It can cause excessive losses of protein, which escapes via the kidneys into the urine. (Normally the urine does not contain substantial amounts of protein.) It also can destroy the white cells of the body.

Because of its potentially serious side effects (summarized in drug table on pp. 204–221), Capoten is reserved for those persons whose essential hypertension cannot be controlled with multiple drugs. It is also used when the side effects of other drugs have proved intolerable, as the effects of Capoten are generally more easily tolerated, though serious as well.

How to Handle Some of the Side Effects

What should you do if you are taking one of these medicines and find yourself suddenly feeling weak, faint, and possibly nauseous to the point of vomiting? Lie down at once with your feet at a level higher than your head. This will help return the blood to your head; the decrease in pressure caused the blood to leave your head. Unless the loss of pressure is extreme, assuming this position should relieve these reactions. If it does not, you will need emergency medical care, including medications, to return your pressure to a better level.

To avoid this situation in the first place, do not stand up or get up suddenly or rapidly when you begin to take these medications. Give yourself a chance to determine how your body reacts to the reduction in pressure. In elderly people, this drop in pressure can be serious, causing complications to the kidney as well as brain damage.

While you are taking any antihypertensive drugs, avoid alcohol, other medications taken without a doctor's permission, strenuous exercise, hot rooms, or a diet too low in salt (unless your doctor has advised it). The new antihypertensive drugs are extremely powerful, and while they can do an outstanding job in reducing many of the complications of hypertension, they also have the potential for serious side effects. You must be under the careful observation of a physician when you take any of these drugs.

A Final Word

It has been the purpose of this book to offer alternate techniques for treating hypertension so that you can avoid the use of drugs or can use a lower dosage, thereby lessening your dependency on medications and your need to deal with side effects. It is important to remember that you can play a part in controlling hypertension—your diet and your life-style can help contribute to the successful treatment of this disorder.

Drug Table

The following drug table is a simplified aid to understanding the various antihypertensive medications and diuretics used in the treatment of hypertension.

Each medication is listed by *brand (or trade) name*—the name given by a particular drug company to its product for the purpose of identification; *generic name*—the chemical or common name used and listed with the Food and Drug Administration; and *company of manufacture*—the company that produces the medication.

The following abbreviations of company names are used:

Abbott—Abbott Pharmaceuticals, Inc.

Ayerst—Ayerst Laboratories

BI—Boehringer Ingelheim Ltd.

Bristol—Bristol Laboratories

Ciba—Ciba Pharmaceutical Company

Geigy—Geigy Pharmaceuticals

HYPERTENSION DRUGS

Glaxo—Glaxo, Inc.

H-R—Hoechst-Roussel Pharmaceuticals, Inc.

Lederle—Lederle Laboratories

Merrell Dow—Merrell Dow Pharmaceuticals, Inc.

MSD—Merck Sharpe & Dohme

Pennwalt—Pennwalt Corporation

Pfizer—Pfizer, Inc.

Robins—A. H. Robins Company

Roche—Roche Laboratories

Sandoz—Sandoz, Inc.

Schering—Schering Corporation

Searle—Searle Pharmaceuticals, Inc.

SKF—Smith Kline and French Laboratories

Squibb—E. R. Squibb & Sons, Inc.

Stuart—Stuart Pharmaceuticals

Upjohn—The Upjohn Company

USV—USV Laboratories, Inc.

Wallace—Wallace Laboratories

Wyeth—Wyeth Laboratories

Following is a list of other antihypertensive agents combined with a diuretic in one formulation:

Aldoclor (MSD)
Aldoril (MSD)
Apresazide (Ciba)
Apresoline-Esidrix (Ciba)
Combipres (BI)
Corzide (Squibb)
Diupres (MSD)
Diutensen (Wallace)
Diutensen-R (Wallace)
Enduronyl (Abbott)
Esimil (Ciba)
Eutron (Abbott)

Hydromox-R (Lederle)
Hydropres (MSD)
Inderide (Ayerst)
Metatensin (Merrell Dow)
Minizide (Pfizer)
Naquival (Schering)
Oreticyl (Abbott)
Rauzide (Squibb)
Renese-R (Pfizer)
Rogroton (USV)
Salutensin (Bristol)

Ser-Ap-Es (Ciba)
Serpasil-Apresoline
  (Ciba)

Serpasil-Esidrix (Ciba)
Tenoretic (Stuart)
Timolide (MSD)

Antihypertensive Medications

Drug Trade Name (Generic Name) and Manufacturer	Action
Aldactazide (hydrochlorothiazide plus spironolactone) Searle	Thiazide diuretic: Increases body fluid loss. Increases output of urine. Causes loss of sodium from the kidney tubules with resultant concomitant loss of water. See Diuril. Potassium-sparing diuretic: Increases urinary output without loss of potassium. See Dyrenium.
Aldactone (spironolactone) Searle	Potassium-sparing diuretic. Acts by inhibiting a specific hormone within the kidneys.
Aldomet (methyldopa) MSD	Antihypertensive. Works in the brain as well as on nerve endings. Decreases renin, the pressure-producing enzyme.

Benefit	Side Effects
Combination diuretic has value not found when either drug is used alone.	Weakness, dizziness, headache, kidney damage, blood problems, increased blood sugar, increased uric acid, other chemical imbalances. Dry mouth, muscle pain, cramps, gastrointestinal upset. See Diuril.
Reduces blood pressure by removing body fluid. Less work for the heart. Less resistance in the vascular system. Less fluid to move.	
Facilitates loss of body fluids but helps retain potassium while allowing sodium to be expelled.	Same as thiazide diuretics; kidney stones, skin rash. See Dyrenium
	Caution: Do not use with other medications unless medically approved.
Has diuretic effect causing loss of potassium.	Same as thiazide diuretics (see Diuril), plus kidney stones, enlarged breasts, impotence, irregular menses, amenorrhea.
	Do not use with other medications unless medically approved.
	Potassium supplements should not be used without a physician's advice.
Long-used agent. Works well when given with thiazide diuretics.	Slows heartbeat, increases stomach acid. Can cause depression, nightmares, liver problems, gastrointestinal upset, flulike symptoms, stuffed nose, drowsiness.

Antihypertensive Medications (continued)

Drug Trade Name (Generic Name) and Manufacturer	Action
Apresoline (hydralazine hydrochloride) Ciba	Works directly on the arteries to reduce resistance, thereby increases rate of flow, reducing internal pressure.
Aquatesen (methyclothiazide) Wallace	Thiazide diuretic. See Diuril.
Blocadren (timolol) MSD	Antihypertensive beta blocker. Acts on receptors in the heart to improve function. Total action not known. Decreases renin. Similar to Tenormin, Corgard, Inderal, Lopressor, Visken.
Bumes (bumetanide) Roche	Loop diuretic. Produces sodium and water loss in kidney tubules (the loop area). Acts in a different area of the kidney than previously known diuretics. Similar diuretic: Lasix.

Benefit	Side Effects
Long-known agent. Works well with other drugs.	Can cause fever, nerve problems, gastro-intestinal upset, head-aches; in some individuals can cause lupus erythematosus.
See Diuril.	See Diuril.
Very effective. High rate of success. Can be used with other agents. Must be used with care in association with other medications.	Asthma, slowed heart-beat, insomnia, impotence, depres-sion, blood problems, heart failure, fatigue, dizziness, confusion, shortness of breath, palpitations, gastro-intestinal complica-tions, rash, itch.
Strong diuretic effect. Can increase dosage until desired results are obtained. Good for hypertensive crisis (severe, sudden onset of hypertension).	Weakness, dizziness, headache, kidney damage, blood problems, increased blood sugar, in-creased uric acid, other chemical imbal-ances, dry mouth, muscle pain, cramps, gastrointestinal upset. Also damage to hearing and ear discomfort. Special care required in pregnancy. May adversely affect fer-tility. Premature ejaculation, difficulty maintaining erection.

Antihypertensive Medications (continued)

Drug Trade Name (Generic Name) and Manufacturer	Action
Capoten (captopril) Squibb	Antihypertensive. Prevents manufacture of renin, the pressure-producing enzyme.
Catapres (clonidine hydrochloride) BI	Antihypertensive, works by blocking the nerve and brain signals that raise blood pressure. Halts renin production.
Corgard (nadolol) Squibb	Antihypertensive beta blocker. See Blocadren.
Diamox (acetazolamide) Lederle	Works to block a specific enzyme in the kidney that controls the outflow of water.
Diuril (chlorothiazide) MSD	Thiazide diuretic. Increases body fluid loss. Increases output of urine. Causes loss of sodium from the kidney tubules with resultant concomitant loss of water.

NOTE: Diuril was one of the first thiazide diuretics used and is

Benefit	Side Effects
Works in conjunction with the usual body mechanisms for controlling elevated blood pressure.	Loss of white blood cells, protein in the urine, gastrointestinal problems.
Can be used in people who have other serious illness such as diabetes, asthma, or heart failure without causing further injury.	Can cause too severe a drop in pressure, rash, fever, flushing, dizziness.
Works well with other diuretic agents.	Dry mouth, gastrointestinal upset, constipation, drowsiness, dizziness, headache, rash, impotence, retention of urine, increased sensitivity to alcohol.
See Blocadren.	See Blocadren.
Produces diuresis by a method different from other diuretics, therefore more valuable in particular situations.	Skin rash, kidney stones, blood problems, tingling in extremities, fever, loss of appetite, imbalance of body chemistry.
Reduces blood pressure by removing body fluids: less work for the heart, less resistance in the vascular system, less fluid to move.	Weakness, dizziness, kidney damage, blood problems, increased blood sugar, increased uric acid, other chemical imbalances, cramps, gastrointestinal upset. Can cause excessive potassium loss.

considered the standard for thiazide diuretics.

Antihypertensive Medications (continued)

Drug Trade Name (Generic Name) and Manufacturer	Action
Dyazide (hydrochlorothiazide plus triamterene) SKF	Thiazide diuretic (see Diuril) and potassium-sparing diuretic (see Dyrenium).
Dyrenium (triamterene) SKF	Potassium-sparing diuretic. Increases urine output but preserves potassium.
Edecrin (ethacrynic acid) MSD	Loop diuretic. See Bumes.
Enduron (methyclothiazide) Abbott	Antihypertensive: Thiazide diuretic. See Diuril.
Esidrix (hydrochlorothiazide) Ciba	Antihypertensive. Thiazide diuretic. See Diuril.

Benefit	Side Effects
See Diuril. See Dyrenium.	See Diuril. See Dyrenium.
Preserves body potassium.	See Diuril; also kidney stones, rash. Do not use with other medications unless medically approved.
Extremely potent diuretic. Used in cases where extreme urinary output is required.	If given in too large a dosage, can cause excessive body loss of water and chemicals. Requires extreme caution. May cause convulsions, loss of appetite, nausea, vomiting, diarrhea, blood problems, dizziness, deafness, rash, headache.
See Diuril.	See Diuril.
See Diuril.	Use with care. See Diuril.

HYPERTENSION DRUGS

Antihypertensive Medications (continued)

Drug Trade Name (Generic Name) and Manufacturer	Action
Eutonyl (pargyline hydrochloride) Abbott	Antihypertensive. Mona-mine-oxidase inhibitor. Blocks the release of nonrepinephrine (adren-aline), which raises body pressure.
Exna (benzthiazide) Robins	Antihypertensive. Thiazide diuretic. See Diuril.
Harmonyl (deserpidine) Abbott	Similar in action to rauwol-fia reserpine. See Rau-dixin.
Hydrodiuril (hydrochlorothiazide) MSD	Antihypertensive. Thiazide diuretic. See Diuril.
Hygroton (chlorthalidone) USV	Thiazide diuretic. See Diuril.
Hylorel (guanadrel sulfate) Pennwalt	Antihypertensive. Blocks nerve action in the blood vessels. Works best with a diuretic.

Benefit	Side Effects
Powerful agent. Used in more severe cases of hypertension.	Can cause shock if one ingests any of the following: foreign beer, Cheddar cheese, yeast, pickled herring, Chianti wine. Also causes headaches, gastrointestinal upset, rash, impotence, retention of urine, dizziness.
See Diuril.	See Diuril.
Useful for use with other antihypertensive as well as alone.	Sedation, insomnia, loss of appetite, impotence, stuffed nose, slowed heart rate, peptic ulcer, severe enough depression to cause suicide.
See Diuril.	See Diuril.
See Diuril.	See Diuril.
Powerful agent, works directly on blood vessels. Works for about eight hours, therefore considered to be short-acting. Easier to control action than for many other antihypertensive agents.	Diarrhea, sexual problems, dizziness, fall in pressure upon standing up, weight gain or loss, blood in urine, insomnia, psychological problems.

Antihypertensive Medications (continued)

Drug Trade Name (Generic Name) and Manufacturer	Action
Hyperstat (diazoxide) Schering	Intravenous antihypertensive agent. Blocks the passage of calcium into the blood vessel walls, causing relaxation and decrease in resistance.
Interal (propranolol hydrochloride) Ayerst	Antihypertensive beta blocker. Acts on receptors in the heart to improve function. Total action is not known. A decrease in blood renin (pressure enzyme) occurs.
Ismelin (guanethidine) Ciba	Antihypertensive. Blocks nerve impulses in the blood vessels. Decreased resistance produces a drop in pressure.
Lasix (furosemide) H-R	Loop diuretic. See Bumes.
Loniten (minoxidil) Upjohn	Direct effect on the blood vessels, decreases resistance. May act by keeping the blood calcium out of the cells.
Lopressor (metoprolol tartrate) Geigy	Antihypertensive beta blocker. See Inderal.

Benefit	*Side Effects*
Powerful agent.	Can only be used intravenously. May cause drop in pressure beyond that wanted. Causes rise in blood sugar, retention of sodium and water, rash, fever, drop in white-cell count.
Effective. Can be used with other agents. No potassium loss. Good control with one-a-day dosage.	Asthma, slowed heartbeat, insomnia, impotence, depression, blood problems, heart failure.
Powerful agent, acts directly on the blood vessels.	Diarrhea, retrograde ejaculation, syncope, loss of pressure upon standing, dry mouth, urinary incontinence, impotence.
See Bumes.	See Bumes
Works well but often requires other drugs in combination. Works in some cases where other combinations do not.	Retention of salt and water, changes in heart function (EKG), hirsutism.
See Inderal.	See Inderal.

Antihypertensive Medications (continued)

Drug Trade Name (Generic Name) and Manufacturer	Action
Lozol (indapamide) USV	Antihypertensive and diuretic. Action not yet understood. Similar to thiazide diuretics with other antihypertensive action.
Maxizide (triamterene plus hydrochloro- thiazide) Lederle	Potassium-sparing thiazide diuretic. See Dyrenium. See Diuril.
Midamor (amiloride hyrochloride) MSD	Potassium-sparing diuretic. Weak action. Similar to Aldactone, Dyrenium.
Minipress (prazosin hydrochloride) Pfizer	Antihypertensive. Proba- bly works as a vasodila- tor, but exact action is not clear. Has blocking action as well.
Moduretic (hydrochlorothiazide plus amilor- ide hydrochloride) MSD	Potassium-sparing thiazide diuretic.
Naqua (trichlormethaizide) Schering	Thiazide diuretic that prevents reabsorption of sodium in the kidneys.
Naturetin (bendroflumethiazide) Squibb	Thiazide diuretic.

Benefit	Side Effects
Long-acting drug needs only one-a-day dosage. Good pressure effects as well as removal of sodium and water.	Mild adverse reactions including headache, dizziness, nervousness, anxiety, gastrointestinal upset, palpitations, urinary frequency, rash, impotence, and reduced libido. Also changes in blood chemistry.
Said to have better proportion of each ingredient, producing better results.	See Dyrenium. See Diuril.
Generally used in combination with thiazide diuretics to save potassium.	See Dyrenium.
Good antihypertensive agent. Can be used alone. Does not interfere with other medications. Does not slow heart or affect blood lipid levels.	Gastrointestinal upset, palpitations, dizziness, blurred vision, rash, impotence, urinary incontinence, stuffed nose.
See Diuril. See Dyrenium.	See Diuril. See Dyrenium.
See Diuril.	See Diuril.
See Diuril.	See Diuril.

Antihypertensive Medications (continued)

Drug Trade Name (Generic Name) and Manufacturer	Action
Normodyne (labetalol hydrochloride) Schering	Antihypertensive. Has two types of nerve blockage: one in the heart and blood vessels and one in the nerves that cause a rise in pressure.
Oretic (hydrochlorothiazide) Abbott	Thiazide diuretic. Prevents reabsorption of sodium in the kidneys. See Diuril.
Procardia (nifedipine) Pfizer	Antihypertensive. Blocks calcium from acting in the cells of the blood vessels.
Raudixin (rauwolfia reserpine) Squibb	Antihypertensive. Blocks nerves that increase blood pressure. Works also on the heart and brain as well as locally on the blood vessels.
Renese (polythiazide) Pfizer	Thiazide diuretic. See Diuril.
Saluron (hydroflumethiazide) Bristol	Thiazide diuretic.
Serpasil (reserpine) Ciba	Antihypertensive. Multiple areas of action, including heart, brain, and blood vessels.

Benefit	Side Effects
Excellent effects without any decrease in kidney function.	Dizziness, tingling, liver changes, asthma, rash, urine retention.
See Diuril.	See Diuril.
Effects reduction in pressure by relaxing the blood vessels.	Can cause too severe a drop in pressure and retention of body water. Also chemical changes in the body, headaches, dizziness, palpitations.
Long-used. One dosage a day.	Sedation, insomnia, loss of appetite, impotence, stuffed nose, slowed heart rate, peptic ulcers, severe enough depression to cause suicide.
See Diuril.	See Diuril.
See Diuril.	See Diuril.
Long-used agent.	Sedation, insomnia, loss of potency, stuffed nose, slowed heart rate, peptic ulcer, severe enough depression to cause suicide.

Antihypertensive Medications (continued)

Drug Trade Name (Generic Name) and Manufacturer	Action
Slow-K (potassium chloride) Ciba	Replaces potassium lost due to medications (diuretics) or due to disease processes.
Tenormin (atenolol) Stuart	Antihypertensive beta blocker.
Trandate (labetalol hydrochloride) Glaxo	Antihypertensive. See Normodyne.
Visken (pindolol) Sandoz	Antihypertensive beta blocker.
Wytensin (guanabenz acetate) Wyeth	Antihypertensive that works in the brain.

Benefit	Side Effects
Helps keep body balanced chemically. Heart, muscles, and nerves will not function if chemistry is imbalanced.	Nausea, vomiting, diarrhea, weakness, confusion, collapse.
See Blocadren.	See Blocadren.
See Normodyne.	See Normodyne.
See Blocadren.	See Blocadren.
Best results when used with a thiazide diuretic, although it works well when used alone.	Dry mouth, gastrointestinal upset, constipation, drowsiness, dizziness, headache, rash, impotence, urinary retention, increased sensitivity to alcohol.

V

MENUS AND RECIPES

~~~~~~

A monthful of low-sodium, low-cholesterol menus for healthful living.

17 ~~~

A Month of Healthy Eating

This chapter contains a month's worth of menus for a 1,200-calorie diet and for a 2,000-calorie diet. The 1,200-calorie diet will help you lose weight; the 2,000-calorie diet will help you maintain your desired weight. Both will allow you to do so while eating well-balanced meals. The recipes referred to in both diet plans appear at the end of this chapter.

All the daily menus contain 1 g or less of sodium and low to moderate amounts of cholesterol. Where possible, the lunch menu suggestions include foods that are available in restaurants or coffee shops. Some minor adjustments may be necessary. If you have a small frame, you may find that 2,000 calories is too much to maintain your desired weight. If so, simply reduce the amount of food you eat daily, but make sure that in doing so you maintain a balanced diet.

NOTE: Where a cooked item is called for, such as

hot cereal, rice, noodles, etc., these should be made without added salt, despite any directions that may be on the box. Finally, asterisks mark items for which recipes are provided—see index for page numbers.

1200-CALORIE DIET
For Weight Loss

Day 1

Breakfast

2 ounces puffed rice (without salt)
½ cup blueberries *or*
   ½ grapefruit
½ cup skim milk
Coffee or tea (optional)

Lunch

Fresh vegetable plate: ½-cup portions of any 4 (raw or
   steamed): asparagus, green beans, broccoli, carrots,
   cauliflower, corn, Brussels sprouts, zucchini
½ cup skim milk
4 ounces green grapes *or*
   1 cup fresh pineapple
Coffee or tea (optional)

Dinner

1 cup Basic Chicken Soup*
¼ recipe Piquant Baked Chicken*
1 cup steamed cauliflower
½ cup cooked brown or white rice
⅓ cup Bittersweet Pudding* *or*
   1 wedge honeydew melon
Coffee or tea (optional)

---

*Asterisks identify items for which recipes are given in this book—see index
for page numbers.

MENUS AND RECIPES

Day 2

Breakfast

½ cup orange juice *or*
   1 cup grapefruit juice
1 egg, poached or otherwise prepared without salt or
   butter
1 slice low-sodium bread
Coffee or tea (optional)

Lunch

1 3-ounce lean, broiled hamburger
1 tomato
1 slice raw onion
½ cup lettuce
½ cup skim milk
½ cup unsweetened applesauce *or*
   1 peach
Coffee or tea (optional)

Dinner

½ cup apple juice
3 Zucchini Boats*
1½ cups lettuce and tomato salad
¼ cup Yogurt Dressing*
1 tangerine *or*
   ½ cup fresh cherries
Coffee or tea (optional)

Day 3

Breakfast

½ cup hot cracked wheat cereal (not instant)
½ cup skim milk
½ grapefruit *or*
    1 peach
Coffee or tea (optional)

Lunch

2 ounces low-sodium Cheddar (or other cheese),
    melted or plain
1 slice low-sodium bread
1 tomato
1 apple *or*
    2 tangerines
Coffee or tea (optional)

Dinner

½ cantaloupe
3 ounces roast turkey (no skin)
⅓ cup cooked noodles sprinkled with poppy seeds
1 cup fresh steamed carrots
1 slice Cheesecake* *or*
    4 ounces green grapes
Coffee or tea (optional)

Day 4

Breakfast

2 ounces puffed wheat (no salt)
½ cup skim milk
½ cantaloupe *or*
    1 banana
Coffee or tea (optional)

Lunch

Curried chicken salad (made with 3 ounces cubed
    chicken, onion, fresh pineapple, curry powder, and
    low-sodium mayonnaise)
Lettuce leaves and cucumber slices
½ cup skim milk
½ grapefruit *or*
    1 apple
Coffee or tea (optional)

Dinner

4 ounces low-sodium tomato juice
4 ounces baked or broiled halibut
½ cup cooked brown or white rice
1 cup Broccoli with Buttermilk Dressing*
1 cup lettuce and tomato salad
1 tablespoon Yogurt Dressing*
1 cup fresh strawberries *or*
    1 nectarine
Coffee or tea (optional)

Day 5

Breakfast

⅔ cup oatmeal (not instant)
½ cup skim milk
1 orange *or*
    ½ cup fresh strawberries
Coffee or tea (optional)

Lunch

Fruit salad plate—½ cup each any 4 fresh
    fruits—grapes, bananas, pears, peaches, plums,
    berries, melons
½ cup low-sodium cottage cheese
1 slice low-sodium bread *or*
    2 breadsticks
Coffee or tea (optional)

Dinner

1 cup Basic Chicken Soup*
¼ recipe Chinese Beef*
½ cup white rice
1 cup steamed zucchini
3 fresh apricots *or*
    1 cup fresh pineapple
Coffee or tea (optional)

MENUS AND RECIPES

Day 6

Breakfast

2 ounces shredded wheat
½ cup skim milk
½ banana *or*
    1 peach
Coffee or tea (optional)

Lunch

3½ ounces broiled, baked, or poached halibut
1 cup steamed broccoli
½ cup steamed carrots
½ cup unsweetened applesauce *or*
    2 plums
Coffee or tea (optional)

Dinner

½ cup Mushroom-Barley Soup*
2 cups Calico Salad*
Raw spinach or lettuce leaves
1 slice Cheesecake* *or*
    1 cup raspberries
Coffee or tea (optional)

Day 7

Breakfast

3 Cottage Cheese Pancakes*
½ cup unsweetened applesauce *or*
    ½ cup blueberries
Coffee or tea (optional)

Lunch

½ recipe Vegetable Salad* or similar combination
¼ cup Yogurt Dressing*
1 apple *or*
    1 pear
½ cup skim milk
Coffee or tea (optional)

Dinner

½ cup marinated mushrooms
3 ounces lean broiled sirloin steak
1 medium baked potato (no butter)
1 cup Broccoli with Buttermilk Dressing*
1 cup mixed salad greens
1 tablespoon Yogurt Dressing*
1 slice Applesauce Cake* *or*
    1 cup watermelon
Coffee or tea (optional)

Day 8

Breakfast

⅔ cup cooked farina made without salt and with skim
   milk instead of water; top with up to 1 teaspoon
   sugar and cinnamon to taste
1 orange *or*
   ½ cantaloupe
Coffee or tea (optional)

Lunch

Pasta salad made with ½ cup cooked pasta and 1 cup
   steamed or raw vegetables
2 tablespoons Oil and Vinegar Dressing* or other
   low-sodium dressing
½ cup skim milk
3 fresh apricots *or*
   ½ cup raspberries
Coffee or tea (optional)

Dinner

½ cup Mushroom-Barley Soup*
¼ recipe Curried Fish*
2 Zucchini Boats*
1 cup lettuce and tomato salad
1 tablespoon Yogurt Dressing*
½ cup Rice Pudding* *or*
   1 wedge honeydew melon
Coffee or tea (optional)

Day 9

Breakfast

2 ounces puffed rice (without salt)
1 cup fresh strawberries *or*
   1 nectarine
½ skim milk
Coffee or tea (optional)

Lunch

3 ounces roast chicken (no skin)
½ cup steamed green beans
½ cup steamed cauliflower
1 banana *or*
   1 apple
Coffee or tea (optional)

Dinner

½ cup Mushroom-Barley Soup*
1 hard-cooked egg
½ recipe Vegetable Salad*
¼ cup Yogurt Dressing*
1 slice Applesauce Cake* *or*
   1 pear
Coffee or tea (optional)

Day 10

Breakfast

1 egg, poached or otherwise prepared without salt or
    butter
1 slice low-sodium bread
½ cup unsweetened applesauce *or*
    1 orange
½ cup skim milk
Coffee or tea (optional)

Lunch

1 cup Basic Chicken Soup* or other low-sodium soup
1 8-ounce carton plain or low-sodium flavored yogurt†
1 banana *or*
    1 cup cherries
Coffee or tea (optional)

Dinner

⅕ recipe Veal with Spaghetti*
1½ cups lettuce and tomato salad
3 tablespoons Yogurt Dressing*
½ cup Rice Pudding* *or*
    1 cup fresh pineapple
Coffee or tea (optional)

†The sodium content of flavored yogurts varies from flavor to flavor and
brand to brand. Read the labels carefully before buying.

Day 11

Breakfast

⅔ cup hot cracked wheat cereal (not instant)
½ cup skim milk
½ grapefruit *or*
   1 peach
Coffee or tea (optional)

Lunch

Fresh vegetable plate: ½-cup portions of any 4 (raw or
   steamed): asparagus, green beans, broccoli, carrots,
   cauliflower, corn, Brussels sprouts, zucchini
½ cup skim milk
4 ounces green grapes *or*
   1 cup fresh pineapple
Coffee or tea (optional)

Dinner

½ cup Mushroom-Barley Soup*
¼ recipe Meat Loaf*
⅓ cup cooked noodles
1 cup fresh green beans, steamed
½ cup Broccoli with Buttermilk Dressing*
2 peaches *or*
   1 pear
Coffee or tea (optional)

Day 12

Breakfast

2 ounces puffed wheat (without salt)
½ cup skim milk
½ cantaloupe *or*
    1 banana
Coffee or tea (optional)

Lunch

1 3-ounce lean hamburger, broiled
1 tomato
1 slice raw onion
½ cup lettuce
½ cup skim milk
½ cup unsweetened applesauce *or*
    1 peach
Coffee or tea (optional)

Dinner

1 cup Basic Chicken Soup*
3 ounces broiled or baked red snapper
1 cup steamed asparagus
1 medium baked potato
1 cup green salad
2 tablespoons Yogurt Dressing*
1 slice Cheesecake* *or*
    1 nectarine
Coffee or tea (optional)

Day 13

Breakfast

⅔ cup oatmeal (not instant)
½ cup skim milk
1 orange *or*
    ½ cup fresh strawberries
Coffee or tea (optional)

Lunch

2 ounces low-sodium Cheddar (or other low-sodium
    cheese), melted or plain
1 slice low-sodium bread
1 tomato
½ cup blueberries *or*
    1 tangerine
Coffee or tea (optional)

Dinner

½ grapefruit
3 ounces lean ground round, broiled
½ cup Eggplant Mélange*
⅓ cup cooked brown or white rice
½ cucumber, peeled, sliced thin, and marinated in
    vinegar
1 slice Applesauce Cake* *or*
    1 cup watermelon
Coffee or tea (optional)

Day 14

Breakfast

2 ounces shredded wheat
½ cup skim milk
½ cup blueberries *or*
   1 peach
Coffee or tea (optional)

Lunch

½ recipe Vegetable Salad* or similar combination
¼ cup Yogurt Dressing*
1 slice low-sodium bread
1 apple *or*
   1 pear
Coffee or tea (optional)

Dinner

1 cup fresh vegetables, raw or steamed, with
2 tablespoons Buttermilk Dressing (see Broccoli with
   Buttermilk Dressing* recipe) as dip
3 ounces lean roast leg of lamb
2 Zucchini Boats*
⅓ cup Bittersweet Pudding* or
   1½ cups watermelon
Coffee or tea (optional)

Day 15

Breakfast

3 Cottage Cheese Pancakes*
½ cup unsweetened applesauce *or*
    ½ grapefruit
½ cup skim milk
Coffee or tea (optional)

Lunch

Pasta salad made with ½ cup cooked pasta and 1 cup
    steamed or raw vegetables
2 tablespoons Oil and Vinegar Dressing* or other
    low-sodium dressing
3 fresh apricots *or*
    1 peach
Coffee or tea (optional)

Dinner

1 cup Basic Chicken Soup*
3 ounces broiled chicken (without skin)
½ cup Eggplant Mélange*
1 cup Broccoli with Buttermilk Dressing*
½ medium baked potato
1 slice Cheesecake* *or*
    1 cup fresh pineapple
Coffee or tea (optional)

Day 16

Breakfast

⅔ cup cooked farina made without salt and with skim
   milk instead of water; top with up to 1 teaspoon
   cinnamon and sugar
1 orange *or*
   ½ cantaloupe
Coffee or tea (optional)

Lunch

Curried chicken salad (made with 3 ounces cubed
   chicken, onion, fresh pineapple, curry powder, and
   low-sodium mayonnaise)
Lettuce and cucumber slices
½ cup skim milk
½ grapefruit *or*
   1 apple
Coffee or tea (optional)

Dinner

1 wedge honeydew melon
¼ recipe Chinese Beef*
½ cup cooked white rice
1 cup steamed zucchini
3 fresh apricots *or*
   1 cup fresh pineapple
Coffee or tea (optional)

Day 17

Breakfast

2 ounces puffed rice (without salt)
½ cup blueberries *or*
    ½ cup grapefruit
½ cup skim milk
Coffee or tea (optional)

Lunch

Fruit salad plate: ½ cup each of any 4 fresh
    fruits—grapes, plums, peaches, bananas, berries
½ cup low-sodium cottage cheese
1 breadstick
Coffee or tea (optional)

Dinner

1 cup Basic Chicken Soup*
¼ recipe Piquant Baked Chicken*
1 cup steamed cauliflower
½ cup steamed fresh peas
½ cup cooked brown or white rice
⅓ cup Bittersweet Pudding* *or*
    1 wedge honeydew melon
Coffee or tea (optional)

Day 18

Breakfast

½ cup orange juice *or*
    1 cup grapefruit juice
1 egg, poached or otherwise prepared without salt or
    butter
1 slice low-sodium bread
½ cup skim milk
Coffee or tea (optional)

Lunch

3½ ounces broiled, baked, or poached halibut
1 cup steamed broccoli
1 medium baked potato
5 dried dates *or*
    1 cup fresh raspberries
Coffee or tea (optional)

Dinner

½ cup low-sodium tomato juice
3 Zucchini Boats*
1½ cups lettuce and tomato salad
¼ cup Yogurt Dressing*
1 wedge honeydew melon *or*
    ½ grapefruit
Coffee or tea (optional)

Day 19

Breakfast

⅔ cup hot cracked wheat cereal (not instant)
½ grapefruit *or*
    1 peach
½ cup skim milk
Coffee or tea (optional)

Lunch

1 cup Basic Chicken Soup* or other low-sodium soup
1 8-ounce carton plain or low-sodium flavored yogurt
1 banana *or*
    1 cup cherries
Coffee or tea (optional)

Dinner

½ cup marinated mushrooms
3 ounces lean sirloin steak, broiled
1 baked potato
1 cup Broccoli with Buttermilk Dressing*
1 cup raw spinach leaves
1 tablespoon Yogurt Dressing*
1 slice Applesauce Cake* *or*
    ½ cantaloupe
Coffee or tea (optional)

Day 20

Breakfast

2 ounces puffed wheat (without salt)
½ cup skim milk
½ cantaloupe *or*
   1 banana
Coffee or tea (optional)

Lunch

3 ounces roast chicken (no skin)
½ cup steamed green beans
½ cup steamed cauliflower
1 pear *or*
   1 cup blackberries
Coffee or tea (optional)

Dinner

½ cup Mushroom-Barley Soup*
¼ recipe Curried Fish*
½ cup Eggplant Mélange*
½ cup cooked brown or white rice
1 cup mixed green salad
1 tablespoon Yogurt Dressing*
⅓ cup Bittersweet Pudding* *or*
   1 wedge honeydew melon
Coffee or tea (optional)

Day 21

Breakfast

⅔ cup oatmeal (not instant)
½ cup skim milk
1 orange *or*
   ½ cup fresh strawberries
Coffee or tea (optional)

Lunch

Pasta salad made with ½ cup cooked pasta and 1 cup
   steamed or raw vegetables
2 tablespoons Oil and Vinegar Dressing* or other
   low-sodium dressing
2 plums *or*
   ½ cup unsweetened applesauce
Coffee or tea (optional)

Dinner

½ cantaloupe
3 ounces roast turkey (no skin)
⅓ cup cooked noodles sprinkled with poppy seeds
1 cup fresh steamed asparagus
½ cup steamed carrots
1 slice Cheesecake* *or*
   4 ounces green grapes
Coffee or tea (optional)

Day 22

Breakfast

2 ounces shredded wheat
½ cup skim milk
½ cup blueberries *or*
    1 peach
Coffee or tea (optional)

Lunch

Fresh vegetable plate—½ cup of any 4, steamed or
    raw: asparagus, green beans, broccoli, cauliflower,
    corn, Brussels sprouts, mushrooms, zucchini
½ cup skim milk
1 cup fresh pineapple *or*
    4 ounces grapes
Coffee or tea (optional)

Dinner

⅕ recipe Veal with Spaghetti*
1½ cups lettuce and tomato salad
3 tablespoons Yogurt Dressing*
½ cup Rice Pudding* *or*
    5 dried dates
Coffee or tea (optional)

Day 23

Breakfast

3 Cottage Cheese Pancakes*
½ cup unsweetened applesauce *or*
    ½ grapefruit
½ cup skim milk
Coffee or tea (optional)

Lunch

1 3-ounce lean hamburger, broiled
1 tomato
1 slice raw onion
½ cup lettuce
1 peach *or*
    1 wedge honeydew melon
Coffee or tea (optional)

Dinner

4 ounces baked or broiled halibut
⅓ cup cooked brown or white rice
1 cup Broccoli with Buttermilk Dressing*
1 cup mixed green salad
1 tablespoon Yogurt Dressing*
⅓ cup Bittersweet Pudding *or*
    1 banana
Coffee or tea (optional)

Day 24

Breakfast

⅔ cup cooked farina, made without salt and with skim
  milk instead of water; top with up to 1 teaspoon
  cinnamon and sugar
1 orange *or*
  ½ cantaloupe
Coffee or tea (optional)

Lunch

2 ounces low-sodium Cheddar or other low-sodium
  cheese, melted or plain
1 slice low-sodium bread
1 tomato
½ cup blueberries *or*
  1 tangerine
Coffee or tea (optional)

Dinner

1 cup Basic Chicken Soup*
2 cups Calico Salad*
Raw spinach or lettuce leaves
1 slice Cheesecake* *or*
  1 pear
Coffee or tea (optional)

Day 25

Breakfast

2 ounces puffed rice (without salt)
½ cup blueberries *or*
   ½ cup grapefruit
½ cup skim milk
Coffee or tea (optional)

Lunch

½ recipe Vegetable Salad* or similar combination
¼ cup Yogurt Dressing*
1 slice low-sodium bread
1 apple *or*
   1 pear
Coffee or tea (optional)

Dinner

½ cup Mushroom-Barley Soup*
¼ recipe Meat Loaf*
⅓ cup cooked noodles
1 cup fresh steamed green beans
½ cup Broccoli with Buttermilk Dressing*
2 peaches *or*
   1 banana
Coffee or tea (optional)

MENUS AND RECIPES
Day 26

Breakfast

½ cup orange juice *or*
  1 cup grapefruit juice
1 egg, poached or otherwise prepared without salt or
  butter
1 slice low-sodium bread
½ cup skim milk
Coffee or tea (optional)

Lunch

Chicken salad (made with 3 ounces cubed chicken and
  low-sodium mayonnaise)
Lettuce and sliced cucumber
½ cup skim milk
½ grapefruit *or*
  1 apple
Coffee or tea (optional)

Dinner

1 cup Basic Chicken Soup* with noodles added
3 ounces broiled or baked red snapper
1 cup steamed asparagus
1 medium baked potato
1 cup mixed green salad
2 tablespoons Yogurt Dressing*
⅓ cup Bittersweet Pudding* *or*
  1 banana
Coffee or tea (optional)

Day 27

Breakfast

2 ounces puffed wheat (without salt)
½ cup skim milk
½ cantaloupe *or*
    1 banana
Coffee or tea (optional)

Lunch

½ cup low-sodium tomato juice
3 ounces roast chicken (no skin)
½ cup steamed green beans
½ cup steamed cauliflower
1 pear *or*
    1 cup blackberries
Coffee or tea (optional)

Dinner

½ grapefruit broiled with ½ tablespoon honey
3 ounces lean ground round, broiled
½ cup Eggplant Mélange*
⅓ cup cooked brown or white rice
½ cucumber, peeled, sliced, and marinated in vinegar
1 slice Applesauce Cake* *or*
    1 nectarine
Coffee or tea (optional)

Day 28

Breakfast

⅔ cup oatmeal (not instant)
½ cup skim milk
1 orange *or*
   ½ cup fresh strawberries
Coffee or tea (optional)

Lunch

1 cup Basic Chicken Soup* or other low-sodium soup
1 8-ounce carton plain or low-sodium flavored yogurt
1 banana *or*
   1 cup cherries
Coffee or tea (optional)

Dinner

1 cup fresh raw or steamed vegetables with
2 tablespoons Buttermilk Dressing* as dip
3 ounces lean roast leg of lamb
2 Zucchini Boats*
1 cup mixed green salad
1 tablespoon Yogurt Dressing*
⅓ cup Bittersweet Pudding* *or*
   1½ cups watermelon chunks
Coffee or tea (optional)

Day 29

Breakfast

2 ounces shredded wheat
½ cup skim milk
½ cup blueberries *or*
    1 peach
Coffee or tea (optional)

Lunch

3½ ounces broiled, baked, or poached halibut
1 cup steamed broccoli
½ cup steamed carrots
1 medium baked potato
3 apricots *or*
    ½ cup fresh raspberries
Coffee or tea (optional)

Dinner

½ cup Mushroom-Barley Soup*
1 hard-cooked egg
½ cup Vegetable Salad*
¼ cup Yogurt Dressing*
⅓ cup Rice Pudding* *or*
    ½ cup unsweetened applesauce
Coffee or tea (optional)

Day 30

Breakfast

⅔ cup cooked farina made without added salt and with
   skim milk instead of water; top with up to 1
   teaspoon cinnamon and sugar
1 orange *or*
   1 peach
Coffee or tea (optional)

Lunch

Fruit salad plate—½ cup each of any 4 fresh fruits:
   grapes, bananas, pears, plums, peaches, berries,
   melons
½ cup low-sodium cottage cheese
1 breadstick
Coffee or tea (optional)

Dinner

1 cup Basic Chicken Soup* with added noodles
3 ounces broiled chicken (no skin)
½ cup Eggplant Mélange*
1 cup Broccoli with Buttermilk Dressing*
¾ cup cooked brown or white rice
1 slice Cheesecake* *or*
   1 cup fresh pineapple
Coffee or tea (optional)

Day 31

Breakfast

3 Cottage Cheese Pancakes*
½ cup unsweetened applesauce *or*
   ½ grapefruit
½ cup skim milk
Coffee or tea (optional)

Lunch

Fresh steamed vegetable plate—½ cup each of any 4,
   steamed or raw: asparagus, beans, broccoli,
   cauliflower, Brussels sprouts, zucchini
½ cup skim milk
4 ounces green grapes *or*
   1 nectarine
Coffee or tea (optional)

Dinner

1 cup low-sodium tomato juice
3 ounces lean sirloin steak, broiled
1 baked potato
1 cup Broccoli with Buttermilk Dressing*
1 cup mixed green salad
1 tablespoon Yogurt Dressing*
1 slice Applesauce Cake* *or*
   ½ cantaloupe
Coffee or tea (optional)

2000-CALORIE DIET
For Maintenance

Day 1

Breakfast

2 ounces puffed rice (without salt)
½ cup blueberries
½ grapefruit
½ cup skim milk
Coffee or tea (optional)

Lunch

Fresh vegetable plate: ½-cup portions of any 4 (raw or
    steamed): asparagus, green beans, broccoli, carrots,
    cauliflower, corn, Brussels sprouts, peas, zucchini
2 ounces Gruyère (or other low-sodium cheese)
1 slice low-sodium bread
1 teaspoon unsalted margarine
½ cup skim milk
4 ounces green grapes *or*
    1 cup fresh pineapple
Coffee or tea (optional)

Dinner

1 cup Basic Chicken Soup* with noodles added
⅓ recipe Piquant Baked Chicken*
1 cup steamed cauliflower
1 cup steamed fresh peas
1 cup cooked brown or white rice
½ cup Bittersweet Pudding* *or*
    1 wedge honeydew melon
Coffee or tea (optional)

258

Day 2

Breakfast

1 cup orange juice *or*
   1 cup grapefruit juice
1 egg, poached or otherwise prepared without salt or
   butter
1 slice low-sodium bread
1 teaspoon unsalted margarine *or*
   1 teaspoon jam or jelly
Coffee or tea (optional)

Lunch

1 4-ounce lean hamburger, broiled
2 slices low-sodium bread
1 tomato
1 slice raw onion
½ cup lettuce
½ cup skim milk
1 nectarine *or*
   5 dried dates
Coffee or tea (optional)

Dinner

½ cup apple juice
3 Zucchini Boats*
1½ cups lettuce and tomato salad
¼ cup Yogurt Dressing* *or*
   3 tablespoons Oil and Vinegar Dressing*
1 ear fresh corn
2 teaspoons unsalted margarine
2 tangerines *or*
   1 cup fresh cherries
Coffee or tea (optional)

Day 3

Breakfast

¾ cup hot cracked wheat cereal (not instant)
1 cup skim milk
1 ounce raisins
½ grapefruit *or*
   1 peach
Coffee or tea (optional)

Lunch

3 ounces low-sodium Cheddar (or other low-sodium
   cheese), melted or plain
2 slices low-sodium bread
1 tomato
1 apple *or*
   2 tangerines
Coffee or tea (optional)

Dinner

½ cantaloupe
4 ounces roast turkey (no skin)
1 cup cooked noodles sprinkled with poppy seeds
1 cup fresh steamed asparagus
½ cup steamed carrots
1 slice low-sodium bread
1 teaspoon unsalted margarine
1 slice Cheesecake* *or*
   6 ounces grapes
Coffee or tea (optional)

Day 4

Breakfast

3 ounces puffed wheat (no salt)
¾ cup skim milk
½ cantaloupe *or*
    1 banana
Coffee or tea (optional)

Lunch

1 cup Mushroom-Barley Soup* or similar low-sodium
    soup
Curried chicken salad (made with 3 ounces cubed
    chicken, onion, fresh pineapple, curry powder, and
    low-sodium mayonnaise)
Lettuce leaves and cucumber slices
2 slices low-sodium bread *or*
    4 breadsticks
2 teaspoons unsalted margarine
½ grapefruit *or*
    1 apple
Coffee or tea (optional)

Dinner

4 ounces low-sodium tomato juice
4 ounces baked or broiled halibut
1 cup cooked brown or white rice
1 cup Broccoli with Buttermilk Dressing*
1 cup lettuce and tomato salad
1 tablespoon Yogurt Dressing* *or*
    1 tablespoon Oil and Vinegar Dressing*
1 cup fresh strawberries *or*
    1 nectarine
Coffee or tea (optional)

Day 5

Breakfast

⅔ cup oatmeal (not instant)
½ cup skim milk
1 orange *or*
    ½ cup orange juice
½ cup fresh strawberries
Coffee or tea (optional)

Lunch

Fruit salad plate—½ cup each of any 4 fresh fruits:
    grapes, bananas, berries, pears, peaches, plums,
    melons
1 cup low-sodium cottage cheese
2 slices low-sodium bread *or*
    4 breadsticks
1 teaspoon unsalted margarine
3 low-sodium cookies
Coffee or tea (optional)

Dinner

1 cup Basic Chicken Soup* with noodles added
⅓ recipe Chinese Beef*
1 cup cooked white rice
1 cup steamed fresh peas
3 fresh apricots *or*
    1 cup fresh pineapple
Coffee or tea (optional)

Day 6

Breakfast

2 ounces shredded wheat
1 cup skim milk
1 banana *or*
   1 peach
Coffee or tea (optional)

Lunch

4 ounces broiled, baked, or poached halibut
1 cup steamed broccoli
½ cup steamed carrots
1 medium baked potato
1 cup unsweetened applesauce *or*
   3 plums
Coffee or tea (optional)

Dinner

1 cup Mushroom-Barley Soup*
2⅓ cups Calico Salad* with chicken if desired
Raw spinach or lettuce leaves
1 slice low-sodium bread
1 teaspoon unsalted margarine
1 slice Cheesecake* *or*
   1 cup raspberries
Coffee or tea (optional)

Day 7

Breakfast

4 Cottage Cheese Pancakes*
1 cup unsweetened applesauce *or*
   1 cup blueberries
Coffee or tea (optional)

Lunch

½ recipe Vegetable Salad* or similar combination
¼ cup Yogurt Dressing* *or*
   3 tablespoons Oil and Vinegar Dressing*
1 slice low-sodium bread
1 teaspoon unsalted margarine
1 apple *or*
   1 pear
½ cup skim milk
Coffee or tea (optional)

Dinner

½ cup marinated mushrooms
4 ounces lean sirloin steak, broiled
1 onion, sautéed in 1 tablespoon oil
1 baked potato
1 cup Broccoli with Buttermilk Dressing*
1 cup mixed salad greens
1 tablespoon Yogurt Dressing* *or*
   1 tablespoon Oil and Vinegar Dressing*
1 slice low-sodium bread
1 teaspoon unsalted margarine
1 slice Applesauce Cake* *or*
   1 cup watermelon
Coffee or tea (optional)

264

Day 8

Breakfast

⅔ cup cooked farina made without salt and with skim
    milk instead of water; top with up to 1 teaspoon
    cinnamon to taste
1 ounce raisins
1 orange *or*
    ½ cantaloupe
Coffee or tea (optional)

Lunch

Pasta salad made with 1 cup cooked pasta and 1½ cups
    raw or steamed vegetables
¼ cup Oil and Vinegar Dressing* or other low-sodium
    dressing
½ cup skim milk
3 fresh apricots *or*
    1 cup raspberries
Coffee or tea (optional)

Dinner

1 cup Mushroom-Barley Soup*
⅓ recipe Curried Fish
2 Zucchini Boats*
1 cup lettuce and tomato salad
1 tablespoon Yogurt Dressing* *or*
    1 tablespoon Oil and Vinegar Dressing*
1 slice low-sodium bread
1 teaspoon unsalted margarine
½ cup Rice Pudding *or*
    1 wedge honeydew melon
Coffee or tea (optional)

Day 9

Breakfast

2 ounces puffed rice (without salt)
1 cup fresh strawberries *or*
    1 nectarine
½ cup skim milk
Coffee or tea (optional)

Lunch

¼ avocado, sliced, with 1 tablespoon Oil and Vinegar
    Dressing* *or*
    3 tablespoons unsalted guacamole
1 breadstick
4 ounces roast chicken (no skin)
½ cup steamed fresh peas
½ cup steamed cauliflower
1 slice low-sodium bread
1 teaspoon unsalted margarine
1 banana *or*
    1 apple
Coffee or tea (optional)

Dinner

1½ cups Mushroom-Barley Soup*
1 hard-cooked egg
½ recipe Vegetable Salad*
¼ cup Yogurt Dressing* *or*
    3 tablespoons Oil and Vinegar Dressing*
1 slice low-sodium bread
1 teaspoon unsalted margarine
1 slice Applesauce Cake* *or*
    1 pear
Coffee or tea (optional)

Day 10

Breakfast

1 egg, poached or otherwise prepared without salt or
    butter
1 slice low-sodium bread
1 teaspoon unsalted margarine
½ cup unsweetened applesauce *or*
    1 orange
½ cup skim milk
Coffee or tea (optional)

Lunch

1 cup Basic Chicken Soup* with added noodles, or
    other low-sodium soup
1 8-ounce carton plain or low-sodium flavored yogurt
1 ear fresh corn
2 breadsticks
1 teaspoon unsalted margarine
1 banana *or*
    1 cup cherries
Coffee or tea (optional)

Dinner

½ cantaloupe
¼ recipe Veal with Spaghetti*
1½ cups lettuce and tomato salad
3 tablespoons Oil and Vinegar Dressing*
2 breadsticks
½ cup Rice Pudding* *or*
    1 cup fresh pineapple
Coffee or tea (optional)

MENUS AND RECIPES
Day 11

Breakfast

1 cup hot cracked wheat cereal (not instant)
1 cup skim milk
½ grapefruit
1 peach
Coffee or tea (optional)

Lunch

Fresh vegetable plate—½ cup portions of any 5 (raw
   or steamed): asparagus, green beans, broccoli,
   carrots, cauliflower, corn, Brussels sprouts, peas,
   zucchini
1 slice low-sodium bread
1 teaspoon unsalted margarine
½ cup skim milk
4 ounces green grapes *or*
   1 cup fresh pineapple
Coffee or tea (optional)

Dinner

1 cup Mushroom-Barley Soup*
⅓ recipe Meat Loaf*
1 cup noodles
1 cup fresh green beans, steamed
1 cup Broccoli with Buttermilk Dressing*
1 slice low-sodium bread
1 teaspoon unsalted margarine
1 slice Applesauce Cake* *or*
   1 pear
Coffee or tea (optional)

268

Day 12

Breakfast

3 ounces puffed wheat (without salt)
¾ cup skim milk
½ cantaloupe *or*
    1 banana
Coffee or tea (optional)

Lunch

1 4-ounce lean hamburger, broiled
2 slices low-sodium bread
1 tomato
1 slice raw onion
½ cup lettuce
½ cup skim milk
1 nectarine *or*
    5 dried dates
Coffee or tea (optional)

Dinner

1 cup Basic Chicken Soup* with added noodles
4½ ounces broiled or baked red snapper
1 cup steamed asparagus
1 medium baked potato
1¼ cups mixed green salad
2 tablespoons Oil and Vinegar Dressing*
1 slice low-sodium bread
1 teaspoon unsalted margarine
1 slice Cheesecake* *or*
    1 pear
Coffee or tea (optional)

Day 13

Breakfast

⅔ cup oatmeal (not instant)
¼ cup skim milk
1 orange
¾ cup fresh strawberries
Coffee or tea (optional)

Lunch

3 ounces low-sodium Cheddar (or other low-sodium
    cheese), melted or plain
2 slices low-sodium bread
1 tomato
1 apple *or*
    2 tangerines
Coffee or tea (optional)

Dinner

½ grapefruit broiled with 1 tablespoon honey
4 ounces lean ground round, broiled
¾ cup Eggplant Mélange*
¾ cup cooked brown or white rice
½ cucumber peeled, sliced, and marinated in vinegar
2 breadsticks *or*
    1 slice low-sodium bread
1 teaspoon unsalted margarine
1 slice Applesauce Cake* *or*
    1 cup watermelon
Coffee or tea (optional)

Day 14

Breakfast

3 ounces shredded wheat
¾ cup skim milk
1 banana *or*
    1 peach
Coffee or tea (optional)

Lunch

½ recipe Vegetable Salad* or similar combination
¼ cup Yogurt Dressing* *or*
    3 tablespoons Oil and Vinegar Dressing*
2 slices low-sodium bread
2 teaspoons unsalted margarine
1 apple *or*
    1 pear
Coffee or tea (optional)

Dinner

1 cup fresh vegetables, raw or steamed, with
2 tablespoons Buttermilk Dressing (see Broccoli with
    Buttermilk Dressing* recipe) as dip
4 ounces lean roast leg of lamb
2 Zucchini Boats*
1 slice low-sodium bread
1 teaspoon unsalted margarine
½ cup Bittersweet Pudding* *or*
    2 cups watermelon
Coffee or tea (optional)

Day 15

Breakfast

4 Cottage Cheese Pancakes*
1 cup unsweetened applesauce
½ grapefruit
⅓ cup skim milk
Coffee or tea (optional)

Lunch

Pasta salad made with 1 cup cooked pasta
   and 1½ cups raw or steamed vegetables
¼ cup Oil and Vinegar Dressing* or other
   low-sodium dressing
2 breadsticks
3 fresh apricots *or*
   1 nectarine
Coffee or tea (optional)

Dinner

1 cup Basic Chicken Soup* with added noodles
4 ounces broiled chicken (without skin)
½ cup Eggplant Mélange*
1 cup Broccoli with Buttermilk Dressing*
1 baked potato
1 slice low-sodium bread
2 teaspoons unsalted margarine
1 slice Cheesecake* *or*
   1 cup fresh pineapple
Coffee or tea (optional)

Day 16

Breakfast

⅔ cup farina made without salt and with skim milk
   instead of water; top with up to 1 teaspoon
   cinnamon and sugar

1 ounce raisins

1 orange *or* ½ cantaloupe

Coffee or tea (optional)

Lunch

1 cup Mushroom-Barley Soup* or similar low-sodium
   soup

Curried chicken salad (made with 3 ounces cubed
   chicken, onion, fresh pineapple, curry powder, and
   low-sodium mayonnaise)

Lettuce and cucumber slices

1 slice low-sodium bread *or* 2 breadsticks

2 teaspoons unsalted margarine

½ cup skim milk

½ grapefruit *or*
   1 apple

Coffee or tea (optional)

Dinner

¼ avocado, sliced, with 1 tablespoon Oil and Vinegar
   Dressing* *or*
   3 tablespoons unsalted guacamole

1 breadstick

⅓ recipe Chinese Beef*

1 cup cooked white rice

1 cup steamed zucchini

3 fresh apricots *or*
   1 cup fresh pineapple

Coffee or tea (optional)

Day 17

Breakfast

2 ounces puffed rice (without salt)
½ cup blueberries
½ grapefruit
1 slice low-sodium bread
1 teaspoon unsalted margarine
½ cup skim milk
Coffee or tea (optional)

Lunch

Fruit salad plate: ½ cup each of any 4 fresh fruits—
    grapes, plums, peaches, bananas, berries, melons
1 cup low-sodium cottage cheese
3 breadsticks
1 teaspoon unsalted margarine
2 low-sodium sugar cookies
Coffee or tea (optional)

Dinner

1 cup Basic Chicken Soup* with added noodles
⅓ recipe Piquant Baked Chicken*
1 cup steamed cauliflower
1 cup steamed fresh peas
1 cup cooked brown or white rice
½ cup Bittersweet Pudding* *or*
    1 wedge honeydew melon
Coffee or tea (optional)

Day 18

Breakfast
½ cup orange juice
1 egg, poached or otherwise prepared without salt or
    butter
1 slice low-sodium bread
1 teaspoon unsalted margarine *or*
    1 teaspoon jam or jelly
½ cup unsweetened applesauce
½ cup skim milk
Coffee or tea (optional)

Lunch
4 ounces broiled, baked, or poached halibut
1 cup steamed broccoli
½ cup steamed carrots
1 medium baked potato
1 slice low-sodium bread
2 teaspoons unsalted margarine
½ cup skim milk
5 dried dates *or* 1 cup fresh raspberries
Coffee or tea (optional)

Dinner
1 cup low-sodium tomato juice *or*
    ½ cup apple juice
3 Zucchini Boats*
1½ cups lettuce and tomato salad
¼ cup Yogurt Dressing* *or*
    3 tablespoons Oil and Vinegar Dressing*
1 ear fresh corn
2 teaspoons unsalted margarine
1 slice Applesauce Cake* *or*
    1 wedge honeydew melon
Coffee or tea (optional)

MENUS AND RECIPES
Day 19

Breakfast

1 cup hot cracked wheat cereal (not instant)
1 cup skim milk
½ grapefruit
1 peach
Coffee or tea (optional)

Lunch

1 cup Basic Chicken Soup* with added noodles, or
    other low-sodium soup
2 breadsticks
1 8-ounce carton plain or low-sodium flavored yogurt
1 ear fresh corn
1 banana *or*
    1 cup cherries
Coffee or tea (optional)

Dinner

½ cup marinated mushrooms
4 ounces lean sirloin steak, broiled
1 sliced onion sautéed in 1 tablespoon oil
1 baked potato
1 cup Broccoli in Buttermilk Dressing*
1 cup raw spinach leaves
1 tablespoon Oil and Vinegar Dressing*
1 slice low-sodium bread
1 teaspoon unsalted margarine
1 slice Applesauce Cake* *or*
    ½ cantaloupe
Coffee or tea (optional)

Day 20

Breakfast

3 ounces puffed wheat (without salt)
¾ cup skim milk
½ cantaloupe
1 banana
Coffee or tea (optional)

Lunch

1 cup low-sodium tomato juice
4 ounces roast chicken (no skin)
½ cup steamed fresh peas
½ cup steamed cauliflower
1 slice low-sodium bread
1 teaspoon unsalted margarine
1 pear *or*
    1 cup blackberries
Coffee or tea (optional)

Dinner

1 cup Mushroom-Barley Soup*
⅓ recipe Curried Fish*
¾ cup Eggplant Mélange
¾ cup cooked brown or white rice
1 cup mixed green salad
1 tablespoon Yogurt Dressing*
1 slice low-sodium bread
1 teaspoon unsalted margarine
½ cup Bittersweet Pudding* *or*
    1 wedge honeydew melon
Coffee or tea (optional)

Day 21

Breakfast

⅔ cup oatmeal (not instant)
1 ounce raisins
¾ cup skim milk
1 orange *or*
   ¾ cup strawberries
Coffee or tea (optional)

Lunch

Pasta salad made with 1 cup cooked pasta and
   1½ cups steamed or raw vegetables
¼ cup Oil and Vinegar Dressing* or other
   low-sodium dressing
2 breadsticks
1 plums *or*
   ½ cup unsweetened applesauce
Coffee or tea (optional)

Dinner

½ cantaloupe
4 ounces roast turkey (no skin)
1 cup cooked noodles sprinkled with poppy seeds
1 cup fresh steamed asparagus
½ cup steamed carrots
1 slice low-sodium bread
1 teaspoon unsalted margarine
1 slice Cheesecake* *or*
   4 ounces green grapes
Coffee or tea (optional)

Day 22

Breakfast

3 ounces shredded wheat
¾ cup skim milk
1 banana *or*
   1 peach
Coffee or tea (optional)

Lunch

Fresh vegetable plate—½ cup of any 5, steamed or
   raw: asparagus, green beans, broccoli, carrots,
   cauliflower, Brussels sprouts, mushrooms, peas,
   zucchini
1 slice low-sodium bread
1 teaspoon unsalted margarine
½ cup skim milk
1 cup fresh pineapple *or*
   4 ounces grapes
Coffee or tea (optional)

Dinner

½ cantaloupe
¼ recipe Veal with Spaghetti*
1½ cups lettuce and tomato salad
3 tablespoons Oil and Vinegar Dressing*
1 breadstick
½ cup Rice Pudding* *or*
   5 dried dates
Coffee or tea (optional)

Day 23

Breakfast

4 Cottage Cheese Pancakes*
½ cup unsweetened applesauce
½ grapefruit
½ cup skim milk
Coffee or tea (optional)

Lunch

1 4-ounce lean hamburger, broiled
2 slices low-sodium bread
1 tomato
1 slice raw onion
½ cup lettuce
½ cup skim milk
1 nectarine *or*
    5 dried dates
Coffee or tea (optional)

Dinner

4 ounces low-sodium tomato juice
4 ounces baked or broiled halibut
1 cup cooked brown or white rice
1 cup Broccoli with Buttermilk Dressing*
1 cup mixed green salad
1 tablespoon Oil and Vinegar Dressing*
½ cup Bittersweet Pudding* *or*
    1 banana
Coffee or tea (optional)

Day 24

Breakfast

⅔ cup cooked farina made without salt and with skim
milk instead of water; top with up to 1 teaspoon
cinnamon and sugar
1 ounce raisins
1 orange *or*
½ cantaloupe
Coffee or tea (optional)

Lunch

3 ounces low-sodium Cheddar (or other low-sodium
cheese), melted or plain
2 slices low-sodium bread
1 tomato
1 apple *or*
2 tangerines
Coffee or tea (optional)

Dinner

1 cup Mushroom-Barley Soup*
2⅓ cups Calico Salad,* with chicken if desired
Raw spinach or lettuce leaves
2 slices low-sodium bread *or*
3 breadsticks
1 teaspoon unsalted margarine
1 slice Cheesecake* *or*
1 pear
Coffee or tea (optional)

Day 25

Breakfast

2 ounces puffed rice (without salt)
½ cup blueberries *or*
    ½ grapefruit
1 slice low-sodium bread
1 teaspoon unsalted margarine *or*
    1 teaspoon jam or jelly
½ cup skim milk
Coffee or tea (optional)

Lunch

1 cup apple juice
½ recipe Vegetable Salad* or similar combination
3 tablespoons Oil and Vinegar Dressing*
2 slices low-sodium bread *or*
    3 breadsticks
2 teaspoons unsalted margarine
1 apple *or*
    1 pear
Coffee or tea (optional)

Dinner

1 cup Mushroom-Barley Soup*
⅓ recipe Meat Loaf*
1 cup cooked noodles
1 cup fresh steamed green beans
1 cup Broccoli with Buttermilk Dressing*
1 slice Applesauce Cake* *or*
    1 banana
Coffee or tea (optional)

Day 26

Breakfast

½ cup orange juice

1 egg, poached or otherwise prepared without salt or
   butter

1 slice low-sodium bread

1 teaspoon unsalted margarine *or*

1 teaspoon jam or jelly

½ cup unsweetened applesauce

½ cup skim milk

Coffee or tea (optional)

Lunch

½ grapefruit broiled with 1 tablespoon honey

Chicken salad made with 3½ ounces cubed chicken
   and low-sodium mayonnaise

Lettuce and sliced cucumber

1 slice low-sodium bread

1 teaspoon unsalted margarine

½ cup skim milk

1 apple *or* 1 nectarine

Coffee or tea (optional)

Dinner

1 cup Basic Chicken Soup* with added noodles

4 ounces baked or broiled red snapper

1 cup steamed asparagus   ½ cup steamed carrots

1 medium baked potato   1 cup mixed green salad

2 tablespoons Yogurt Dressing* *or*
     2 tablespoons Oil and Vinegar Dressing*

1 slice low-sodium bread

1 teaspoon unsalted margarine

½ cup Bittersweet Pudding* *or*
     1 banana

Coffee or tea (optional)

Day 27

Breakfast

3 ounces puffed wheat (without salt)
¾ cup skim milk
½ cantaloupe *or*
   1 banana
Coffee or tea (optional)

Lunch

1 cup low-sodium tomato juice
4 ounces roast chicken (no skin)
½ cup steamed fresh peas
½ cup steamed cauliflower
1 slice low-sodium bread
1 teaspoon unsalted margarine
1 pear *or*
   1 cup blackberries
Coffee or tea (optional)

Dinner

½ grapefruit broiled with 1 tablespoon honey
4 ounces broiled lean ground round
¾ cup Eggplant Mélange*
1 cup cooked brown or white rice
½ cucumber peeled, sliced, and marinated in vinegar
1 slice low-sodium bread
1 teaspoon unsalted margarine
1 slice Applesauce Cake* *or*
   1 nectarine
Coffee or tea (optional)

Day 28

Breakfast

⅔ cup oatmeal (not instant)
1 ounce raisins
¾ cup skim milk
1 orange *or*
   ¾ cup fresh cherries
Coffee or tea (optional)

Lunch

1 cup Basic Chicken Soup* with added noodles, or
   other low-sodium soup
2 breadsticks
1 8-ounce carton plain or low-sodium flavored yogurt
1 ear fresh corn
1 banana *or*
   1 cup cherries
Coffee or tea (optional)

Dinner

1 cup fresh raw or steamed vegetables with
2 tablespoons Buttermilk Dressing (see Broccoli with
   Buttermilk Dressing* recipe) as dip
4 ounces lean roast leg of lamb
2 Zucchini Boats*
1½ cups mixed green salad
2 tablespoons Oil and Vinegar Dressing*
1 slice low-sodium bread
1 teaspoon unsalted margarine
½ cup Bittersweet Pudding* *or*
   2 cups watermelon chunks
Coffee or tea (optional)

Day 29

Breakfast

3 ounces shredded wheat
¾ cup skim milk
1 banana *or*
   1 peach
Coffee or tea (optional)

Lunch

4 ounces broiled, baked, or poached halibut
1 cup steamed broccoli
½ cup steamed carrots
1 medium baked potato
1 slice low-sodium bread
2 teaspoons unsalted margarine
5 dried dates *or*
   1 cup fresh raspberries
Coffee or tea (optional)

Dinner

1 cup Mushroom-Barley Soup*
1 hard-cooked egg
½ recipe Vegetable Salad*
¼ cup Yogurt Dressing*
1 ear fresh corn
1 slice low-sodium bread
2 teaspoons unsalted margarine
½ cup Rice Pudding* *or*
   ½ cup unsweetened applesauce
Coffee or tea (optional)

Day 30

Breakfast

⅔ cup cooked farina made without salt and with skim
    milk instead of water; top with up to 1 teaspoon
    cinnamon and sugar
1 ounce raisins
1 orange *or*
    1 peach
Coffee or tea (optional)

Lunch

Fruit salad plate—½ cup each of any 4 fresh fruits:
    grapes, bananas, pears, peaches, berries, melons
1 cup low-sodium cottage cheese
3 breadsticks
1 teaspoon unsalted margarine
2 low-sodium cookies
Coffee or tea (optional)

Dinner

1¼ cups Basic Chicken Soup* with added noodles
4 ounces broiled chicken (no skin)
½ cup Eggplant Mélange
1 cup Broccoli with Buttermilk Dressing*
1 cup cooked brown or white rice
1 slice low-sodium bread
1 teaspoon unsalted margarine
1 slice Cheesecake* *or*
    1 cup fresh pineapple
Coffee or tea (optional)

Day 31

Breakfast
4 Cottage Cheese Pancakes*
½ cup unsweetened applesauce
½ grapefruit
½ cup skim milk
Coffee or tea (optional)

Lunch
Fresh vegetable plate—any 4, steamed or raw:
    asparagus, beans, broccoli, cauliflower, Brussels
    sprouts, peas, carrots, zucchini
1 slice low-sodium bread
1 teaspoon unsalted margarine
½ cup skim milk
4 ounces green grapes *or*
    1 nectarine
Coffee or tea (optional)

Dinner
1 cup low-sodium tomato juice
4 ounces lean sirloin steak, broiled
1 sliced onion, sautéed in 1 tablespoon oil
1 baked potato
1 cup Broccoli in Buttermilk Dressing*
1½ cups mixed green salad
2 tablespoons Yogurt Dressing* *or*
    2 tablespoons Oil and Vinegar Dressing*
1 slice low-sodium bread
1 teaspoon unsalted margarine
1 slice Applesauce Cake* *or*
    ½ cantaloupe
Coffee or tea (optional)

RECIPES

Basic Chicken Soup

3 pounds chicken, cut up
3 quarts water
1 cup chopped onion
1 stalk celery, chopped
3 carrots, peeled and sliced
2 cloves garlic, minced
1 parsnip, chopped (optional)
3 sprigs parsley (preferably flat-leaf)
1 bay leaf
Black pepper, freshly ground, to taste

Clean the chicken and discard any visible fat. Place in a large, heavy pot. Add all the remaining ingredients and bring to a boil. Skim if necessary. Lower the heat and simmer uncovered, stirring occasionally, for 2¼ hours.

For *Basic Chicken Stock*, let the liquid cool and then strain. Discard the bay leaf and parsley. Refrigerate the stock until any fat congeals, and then discard fat.

The strained bouillon can be refrigerated or frozen and used as needed.

For Basic Chicken Soup, to the stock add 1½ cups of the cooked chicken, skin removed, diced, with skin and bones discarded (use the remaining chicken for other recipes), the cooked vegetables, 3 tablespoons chopped green pepper, and 2 tablespoons minced parsley. Two to 6 ounces of fine noodles may also be added. Heat through until added ingredients are tender, and serve.

Makes 10 cups.

Mushroom-Barley Soup

2 tablespoons corn or safflower oil
2 onions, sliced
1 clove garlic, minced
¾ pound fresh mushrooms, sliced
1 carrot, peeled and diced
1 bay leaf
¼ cup pearled barley
4 cups Basic Chicken Stock (see Basic Chicken Soup* recipe)
1 tablespoon cornstarch
½ cup skim or low-fat milk
1 tablespoon lemon juice
2 tablespoons minced parsley

Heat the oil in the bottom of a large, heavy pot. Add the onion and garlic and sauté until the onion is translucent, about 5 minutes. Add the mushrooms, and sauté for 5 more minutes.

Add the carrot, bay leaf, barley, and stock to the pot. Bring to a boil, cover, and simmer over low heat for 50 minutes.

Stir the cornstarch into the milk with a wire whisk and stir until free of lumps. Add a small amount of hot soup to the mixture and then stir all the milk mixture into the soup. Add the lemon juice and stir well. Reheat but do not boil. Serve sprinkled with parsley.

Makes about 5 cups.

Vegetable Salad

4 cups Boston or Romaine lettuce (or use half lettuce, half raw spinach)
1 green pepper, seeded and cut into julienne strips
1 cup broccoli, steamed until just tender and cooled
1 tomato, cut into eighths
½ small onion, sliced into thin rings
½ cup fresh peas, raw or lightly steamed
1 cucumber, peeled and sliced thin

Combine all ingredients in a salad bowl and toss gently. Serve with Yogurt Dressing* or Oil and Vinegar Dressing*

Makes about 6 cups.

Calico Salad

3 cups cooked brown or white rice (cooked without salt)
1 carrot, peeled and diced
1 stalk broccoli, chopped
1 medium zucchini, about ½ pound
¼ cup onion, chopped fine, *or* 2 scallions, chopped
2 tablespoons red or green pepper, chopped
1 tablespoon minced parsley
1 cup diced roast chicken or turkey, without skin (optional)
1 tablespoon tarragon vinegar
1 tablespoon lemon juice
1 large clove garlic, minced
¾ teaspoon dry mustard
¼ cup corn or safflower oil

Place the rice in a large bowl.

Steam the carrots and broccoli until just tender and add to the rice. Add the zucchini, onion, pepper, and parsley. Add the chicken or turkey, if desired, and stir until well mixed.

291

Stir the vinegar, lemon juice, garlic, and mustard with a wire whisk. Beat in the oil gradually. Pour over the rice mixture and stir gently until all is coated. Let salad marinate at room temperature for 2 hours. Serve at room temperature, surrounded by lettuce or spinach leaves.

Makes 6 to 7 cups.

Meat Loaf

1 pound lean ground beef (or use ½ pound beef and ½ pound ground veal)
1 medium onion, finely chopped
1 clove garlic, minced
¼ cup low-sodium bread crumbs† or
    ¼ cup rolled oats (not instant)
¼ cup chopped fresh parsley (preferably flat-leaf)
½ cup Tomato Sauce*
Preheat oven to 350°F.

Mix the meat, onion, garlic, crumbs, parsley, and ¼ cup tomato sauce together well. Shape into a loaf and place in a pan. Bake at 350°F for 45 minutes.

Pour the reserved ¼ cup tomato sauce over the top and bake an additional 15 minutes.

Serves 3 to 4.

*To make low-sodium bread crumbs, place a few slices of low-sodium bread (slightly stale is fine) in food processor. Process until you have fine crumbs. Keep in refrigerator or freezer and use as needed.

Tomato Sauce

1 tablespoon corn oil or safflower oil
1 medium onion, chopped
2 cloves garlic, minced
2 tomatoes, skins removed†
2 8-ounce cans no-salt-added tomato sauce
½ cup water
1 tablespoon fresh parsley (preferably flat-leaf), minced
½ teaspoon basil
1 teaspoon oregano

Heat the oil in a large skillet. Add the onion and garlic and sauté until onion is golden.

Chop the tomatoes. Stir the tomatoes, tomato sauce, water, parsley, basil, and oregano into the onion mixture.

Bring to a boil, cover, and simmer over low heat, stirring occasionally, for 30 minutes.

Makes about 2½ cups.

Chinese Beef

1 pound flank steak
2 tomatoes
1 green pepper, seeded
1 red pepper, seeded
2 tablespoons corn oil or safflower oil
1 onion, sliced thin
1 cup mushrooms, sliced
1 clove garlic, minced
3 tablespoons sherry
¼ teaspoon ground ginger
2 tablespoons lemon juice
1 tablespoon sugar
1 tablespoon cornstarch
¼ cup water

†To remove skins from tomatoes, dip into boiling water for about 20 seconds. Skins will slip off easily.

Cut the flank steak across the grain into thin strips.

Cut the tomatoes and peppers into 2-inch chunks.

Heat the oil in a wok or large skillet. Add the beef and stir over high heat until browned, about 5 minutes.

Remove the beef from the wok with a slotted spoon. Add the tomatoes, peppers, onion, mushrooms, and garlic to the wok. Stir over high heat until peppers are barely tender, about 3 minutes.

Return the beef to the pan. Add the sherry, ginger, lemon juice, and sugar. Bring to a boil, cover, and cook over low heat for 3 minutes.

Make a smooth paste of the cornstarch and water. Stir into the beef mixture and cook 2 minutes, or until sauce is thickened. Serve with rice.

Serves 4 to 5.

Veal with Spaghetti

1 pound ground veal
¼ cup low-sodium bread crumbs (see footnote on page 239)
¼ cup skim or low-fat milk
2 tablespoons minced parsley
1 clove garlic, minced
Black pepper, freshly ground, to taste
1 tablespoon corn oil
2 green peppers, seeded and cut into julienne strips
⅓ pound mushrooms, sliced
1 onion, sliced thin
1 clove garlic (additional), minced
1 teaspoon dried basil
½ teaspoon dried oregano
1 14½-ounce can no-salt-added stewed tomatoes
2 8-ounce cans no-salt-added tomato sauce
⅓ cup water
½ pound spaghetti, cooked without salt

Mix the veal, bread crumbs, milk, parsley, garlic, and pepper together well. Shape into small meatballs about 1 inch in diameter. There should be 25 to 30 meatballs.

Heat the oil in a large skillet. Add the meatballs and sauté, turning gently, until lightly browned. Remove with a slotted spoon and set aside. Add the peppers, mushrooms, onion, and garlic to the pan and sauté until the onion is translucent.

Return the meatballs to the pan. Stir in the basil, oregano, stewed tomatoes, tomato sauce, and water. Simmer, uncovered, over low heat for 15 minutes, stirring often.

Pour veal and sauce over hot cooked spaghetti, toss gently, and serve with a green salad.

Serves 4 to 6.

Piquant Baked Chicken

2½ pounds chicken breasts
3 tablespoons water
⅓ cup fresh lemon juice
½ teaspoon dry mustard
¼ teaspoon garlic powder
1 teaspoon onion powder
½ teaspoon black pepper, freshly ground
⅓ cup low-sodium bread crumbs (see footnote on page 292)
2 teaspoons minced parsley

Preheat oven to 350°F.

Remove the skin and all visible fat from chicken and discard.

Mix the water, lemon juice, dry mustard, garlic and onion powders, and pepper together well. Add the chicken and marinate for 1 hour.

Mix the bread crumbs and parsley on a flat plate. Dip the marinated chicken pieces in the crumb mixture and arrange in a shallow baking pan large enough to hold all the pieces in one layer.

Bake at 350°F for 45 minutes to 1 hour, or until tender.

Serves 4.

Curried Fish

¼ cup no-salt-added cottage cheese
¼ cup no-salt-added farmer cheese
3 tablespoons plain yogurt
½ teaspoon curry powder
1 teaspoon lemon juice
1 pound flounder fillets

Preheat oven to 350°F.

Mix the cottage cheese, farmer cheese, yogurt, curry powder, and lemon juice with a wire whisk until smooth.

Arrange the fish in one layer in a shallow baking pan. Spoon the curry mixture over the fish. Bake at 350°F 20 to 30 minutes, until fish flakes easily with a fork. Do not overcook.

Serves 3 to 4.

Zucchini Boats

6 zucchini, about ½ pound each
2 tablespoons corn or safflower oil
1 onion, chopped
1 stalk celery, chopped
2 cloves garlic, minced
½ pound mushrooms, sliced
1 carrot, peeled and shredded
2 tablespoons green pepper, chopped
2 cups cooked brown or white rice (cooked without salt)
1 14½ ounce can no-salt-added stewed tomatoes, drained,
   with liquid reserved
2 tablespoons minced parsley
½ teaspoon basil
Black pepper, freshly ground, to taste

Wash the zucchini and cut off stem ends. Drop in boiling water and cook, uncovered, for 7 minutes. Drain and cut in half lengthwise. Scoop out pulp with a spoon and set shells aside. Chop the pulp.

Heat the oil in a skillet. Add the onion, celery, and garlic. Sauté until the onion is translucent, about 5 minutes. Add the zucchini pulp, mushrooms, carrot, and green pepper to the pan. Sauté until the mushrooms give up their liquid, about 5 minutes.

Turn into a large mixing bowl. Add the rice, tomatoes, parsley, basil, and pepper. Stir gently until well mixed. Spoon evenly into the 12 zucchini shells.

Spray one or two shallow baking dishes with no-salt-added, low-calorie vegetable coating and arrange shells in a single layer.

Bake at 350°F for 40 minutes, basting occasionally with the reserved tomato liquid. Serve with a green salad as a main dish or as a vegetable side dish.

Serves 4 as a main dish, 6 as a side dish.

Eggplant Mélange

1 medium eggplant, about 1½ pounds
1 stalk celery, chopped
1 onion, chopped
2 cloves garlic, chopped
4 tablespoons chopped green pepper
1 14½ ounce can no-salt-added stewed tomatoes

Wash eggplant, remove stem end, and cut into ¾-inch cubes.

Spray a large skillet with no-salt-added, vegetable low-calorie spray. Heat, then add the eggplant cubes, celery, onion, and garlic. Sauté, stirring frequently, over medium-high heat, for 10 minutes.

Add the green pepper and stewed tomatoes and their liquid to skillet. Cook, uncovered, for about 2 minutes, or until all is tender.

Makes about 4 cups.

Broccoli with Buttermilk Dressing

2 tablespoons low-fat, no-salt-added buttermilk
2 tablespoons plain yogurt
3 tablespoons no-salt-added farmer cheese
1 clove garlic
2 teaspoons onion
1 tablespoon fresh parsley
1 bunch broccoli

To make *Buttermilk Dressing*: Place all ingredients, except broccoli, in the container of a food processor or blender. Process until smooth.

Steam the broccoli until tender. Turn into a bowl and spoon on dressing. Serve hot or chilled.

Makes ⅔ cup dressing, 4 cups broccoli.

NOTE: The dressing is also good as a dip for raw vegetables.

Yogurt Dressing

½ cup plain yogurt
½ cucumber, peeled, seeded, and cut into chunks
1 small clove garlic, minced
1 tablespoon minced onion
1 tablespoon minced fresh parsley
¼ cup no-salt-added, low-fat cottage cheese
1 teaspoon lemon juice

Place all the ingredients in the container of a food processor or blender. Process until smooth.

Store in refrigerator in a screw-top jar. Shake before using. Will keep at least 2 weeks in refrigerator.

Makes about 1¾ cups.

Oil and Vinegar Dressing

¼ cup tarragon vinegar
½ teaspoon dry mustard
Black pepper, freshly ground, to taste
1 clove garlic, minced
1 teaspoon minced parsley
1 teaspoon minced onion or scallion
½ teaspoon sugar
½ cup corn or safflower oil

Beat the vinegar, mustard, pepper, garlic, parsley, onion, and sugar together with a wire whisk. Beat the oil in slowly, a little at a time, until well blended.

Store in refrigerator in a screw-top jar, and shake well before using. Keeps at least 2 weeks in refrigerator. Use on salads and as a marinade for vegetables and lean meats.

Makes ¾ cup.

NOTE: Red-wine vinegar and/or lemon juice may be used in place of the tarragon vinegar.

Cottage Cheese Pancakes

1 egg
1 cup no-salt-added, low-fat cottage-cheese
⅔ cup flour
1 tablespoon corn oil or safflower oil
½ cup low-fat milk

Beat the egg in a medium-sized bowl. Add the cottage cheese, flour, oil, and milk. Stir until well mixed.

Spray a griddle or large skillet with no-salt-added, low-calorie vegetable spray. Heat the griddle, and then drop batter by the spoonful onto hot griddle. Use about 2 tablespoons batter per pancake.

Cook until bottoms are lightly browned and pancake tops are bubbly. Turn and brown other side.

Serve lightly sprinkled with cinnamon and sugar, or with applesauce or fresh fruit.

Makes about 10 pancakes.

Applesauce Cake

2 eggs, separated
1 cup sugar
⅓ cup skim or low-fat milk
⅓ cup apple juice
3 tablespoons fresh lemon juice
2 teaspoons cinnamon
¼ teaspoon nutmeg
1 teaspoon vanilla
1 15-ounce jar unsweetened applesauce
1⅓ cups sifted flour

Preheat oven to 350°F.

Spray a 10-inch springform pan with no-salt added, low-calorie vegetable spray, or oil lightly with corn oil or safflower oil. Set aside.

Beat the egg yolks slightly in the bowl of an electric mixer. Add the sugar gradually in a steady stream until mixture is thick and lemon-colored. Beat in the milk, apple juice, lemon juice, cinnamon, nutmeg, and vanilla. Add the applesauce and flour alternately, a little at a time, until both are used up.

Beat the egg whites until stiff. Fold gently into the applesauce mixture. Pour batter into prepared pan.

Bake at 350°F for 35 to 40 minutes, or until a toothpick inserted in middle comes out clean.

Makes 1 10-inch cake; serves 12.

Cheesecake

⅓ cup low-sodium bread crumbs (see footnote on page 292)
1 7½-ounce package no-salt-added farmer cheese
1 cup low-fat, no-salt-added cottage cheese
1 envelope unflavored gelatin
¼ cup apple juice
2 eggs, separated
½ cup skim or low-fat milk
½ cup sugar
2 tablespoons lemon juice
1 teaspoon vanilla

Line the bottom of an 8-inch springform pan with the bread crumbs. Set aside.

Beat the farmer cheese and cottage cheese with an electric mixer until very smooth. Set aside.

Sprinkle the gelatin over the apple juice and set aside to soften.

Beat the egg yolks in the top of a double boiler. Add the milk and sugar, and stir over simmering water until the mixture thickens, about 10 minutes. Stir in the gelatin-apple-juice mixture and cool over a bowl of ice cubes or in the refrigerator.

Beat the cooled custard mixture until smooth, then add the cheese mixture, lemon juice, and vanilla. Beat the egg whites until stiff, and fold in gently. Pour the mixture into the prepared pan, and chill until firm.

Makes 1 8-inch cake; serves 10.

Rice Pudding

1 cup apple juice
1 cup low-fat milk
3 tablespoons sugar
1 teaspoon vanilla
1 teaspoon cinnamon
1 teaspoon lemon juice
2 cups cooked rice (cooked without salt)

Preheat oven to 325°F.

Mix the apple juice, milk, sugar, vanilla, cinnamon, and lemon juice together well. Stir in the rice.

Spray a baking dish with no-salt-added, low-calorie vegetable spray. Pour in the rice mixture and bake at 325°F for 50 minutes, or until set.

Makes about 3 cups.

Bittersweet Pudding

¾ cup low-fat milk
3 tablespoons cornstarch
½ cup sugar
3 tablespoons unsweetened cocoa
1 cup low-fat, no-salt-added buttermilk
¼ cup black coffee
1 teaspoon vanilla
½ teaspoon almond extract

Mix ¼ cup of the low-fat milk with the cornstarch. Stir with a wire whisk until completely smooth and free of any lumps. Set aside.

Place the sugar, cocoa, buttermilk, coffee, and remaining ½ cup low-fat milk in the top of a double boiler. Place over simmering water and cook, stirring, until warmed through. Add the cornstarch mixture and stir over barely boiling water until thickened, about 10 minutes. Stir in the vanilla and almond extracts.

Turn into a serving bowl or individual dishes, and chill until firm.

Makes 2 cups; serves 4 to 6.

Appendix

Sources for Help with Alcohol and Tobacco

For alcohol:
    National Clearinghouse for Alcohol Information
    1776 East Jefferson South, 4th Floor
    Rockville, MD 20852 *or*
    P.O. Box 2345
    Rockville, MD 20850

For tobacco:
    Technical Information Center
    Office on Smoking and Health
    5600 Fishers Lane, Room 1–16
    Rockville, MD 20857

Biofeedback Information

    Francine Butler, Ph.D.
    Biofeedback Society of America
    University of Colorado Medical Center, C268
    4200 East Ninth Avenue
    Denver, CO 80262

Newsletters:
Biofeedback Network
Dub Rakestraw, Editor
103 South Grove
Greenburg, KS 67054

Brain/Mind Bulletin
M. Ferguson, Editor
P.O. Box 42211
Los Angeles, CA 90004

Bibliography

General Publications on Hypertension and Its Management

Alcohol and Health: Fifth Special Report to the U.S. Congress from the Secretary of Health and Human Services, December 1983. Washington, D.C.: U.S. Department of Health and Human Services. Public Health Service, DHHs Pub. No. (ADM) 84-12, 1984.

Modern Drug Encyclopedia, 16th ed. Arthur J. Lewis, M.D., ed. New York: Yorke Medical Books, 1981.

1980 Report of the Joint National Committee on Detection, Evaluation, and Treatment of High Blood Pressure. Bethesda, Md.: National Heart, Lung, and Blood Institute, National Institutes of Health. Pub. No. 81-1088, 1980.

Physicians' Desk Reference, 39th ed. Oradell, N.J.: Medical Economics Company, 1985.

Dawber, T. R. *The Framingham Study*. Cambridge, Mass.: Harvard University Press, 1980.

Farquhar, J. W. *The American Way of Life Need Not Be Hazardous to Your Health*. New York: Norton, 1979.

Friedman, Meyer, and Rosenman, Ray. *Type A Behavior and Your Heart*. New York: Alfred A. Knopf, 1974.

Kaplan, Norman. *Clinical Hypertension*. Baltimore, Md.: The Williams & Wilkins Company, 1982.

Selye, Hans. *Stress Without Distress*. New York: Harper & Row, 1974.

Measuring the Sodium and Cholesterol in Your Diet

Kraus, Barbara. *The Dictionary of Sodium, Fats, and Cholesterol*. New York: Grosset & Dunlap, 1979.

———. *The Barbara Kraus Guide to Sodium*. New York: Signet Books, 1983.

Information on Medications and Their Side Effects

Graedon, Joe. *The People's Pharmacy*. New York: Avon Books, 1976.

———. *The People's Pharmacy—Two*. New York: Avon Books, 1980.

Krupp, Marcus A., et al. *Current Medical Diagnosis and Treatment*. Los Angeles, Calif.: Lange Medical Publications, 1985.

Modern Drug Encyclopedia, 16th ed. Arthur J. Lewis, M.D., ed. New York: Yorke Medical Books, 1981.

Physicians' Desk Reference, 39th ed. Oradell, N.J.: Medical Economics Company, 1985.

Cookbooks That Will Help You Eat Right

DeBakey, Michael, et al. *The Living Heart Diet*. New York: Simon & Schuster, 1985.

Eshelman, Ruthe, and Winston, Mary. *The American Heart Association Cookbook*. New York: Ballantine Books, 1980.

Margie, Joyce D., and Hunt, James C. *Living with High Blood Pressure: The Hypertensive Diet Cookbook*. Radnor, Pa.: Chilton, 1979.

Bibliography

Roth, Harriet. *Deliciously Low: The Gourmet Guide to Low-Sodium, Low-Fat, Low-Cholesterol, Low-Sugar Cooking*. New York: Plume Books, 1984.

Schell, Merle. *Tasting Good: The International Salt-Free Diet Cookbook*. New York: Plume Books, 1982.

Stead, Evelyn S., and Warren, Gloria K. *Low-Fat Cookery*. New York: McGraw-Hill, 1977.

Stern, Ellen, and Michaels, Jonathan. *The Good Heart Diet Cookbook*. New York: Ticknor & Fields, 1982.

Waldo, Myra. *The Low-Salt, Low-Cholesterol Cookbook*. New York: Berkley, 1982.

INDEX

Index

About the Author

Robert L. Rowan, M.D., F.A.C.S., is a Clinical Associate Professor at New York University Medical School in New York City. He has co-authored two previous books and has contributed many scientific articles to medical literature.